THE A TO ZEN OF YOGA

HOW TO GET RID OF EMOTIONAL BAGGAGE BY TOUCHING YOUR TOES....

Sarah Tucker

Published by New Generation Publishing in 2015

Copyright © Sarah Tucker 2015

First Edition

The author asserts the moral right under the Copyright, Designs and Patents Act 1988 to be identified as the author of this work.

All Rights reserved. No part of this publication may be reproduced, stored in a retrieval system or transmitted, in any form or by any means without the prior consent of the author, nor be otherwise circulated in any form of binding or cover other than that which it is published and without a similar condition being imposed on the subsequent purchaser.

www.newgeneration-publishing.com

 New Generation Publishing

Always for Tom

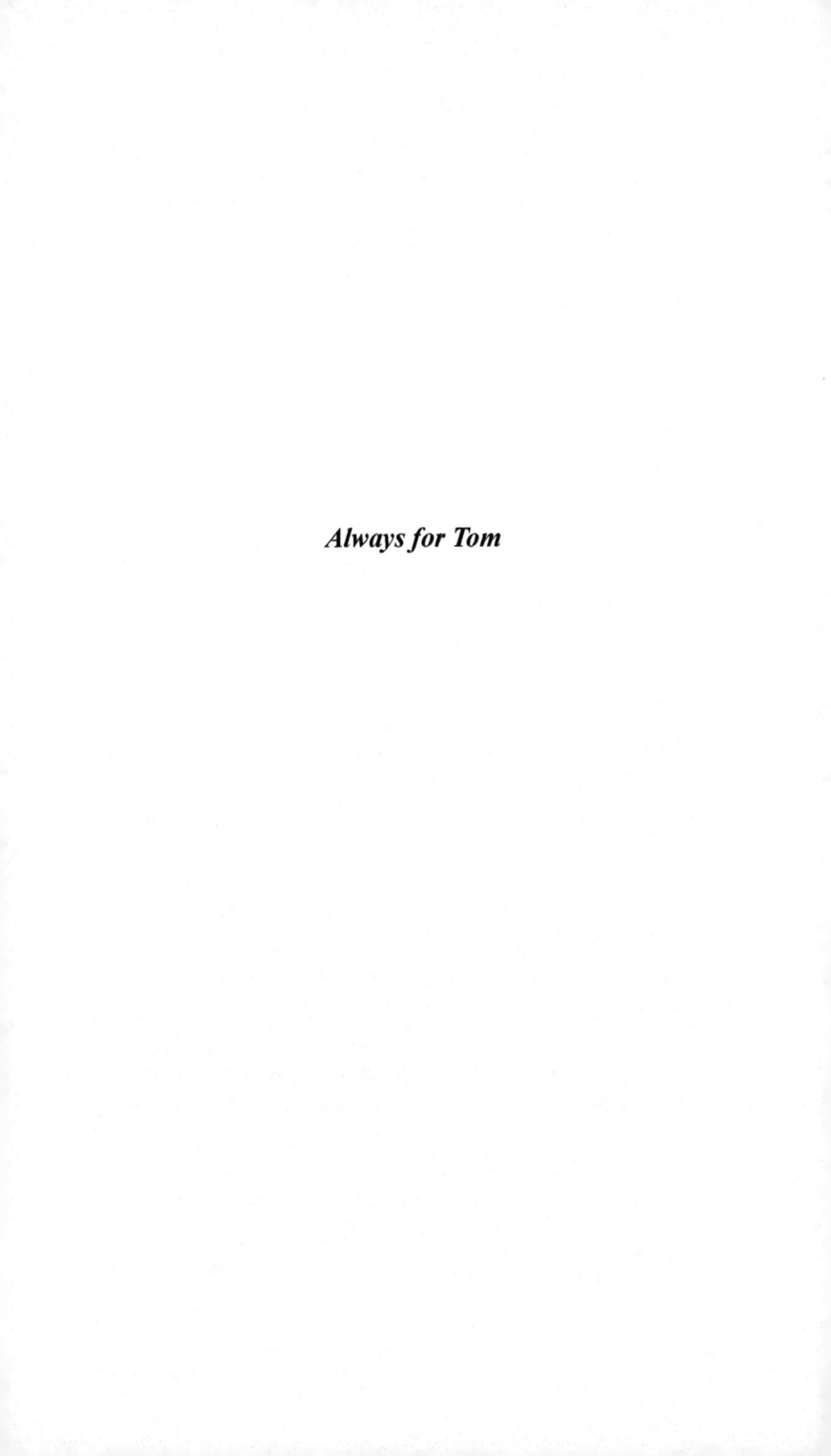

Introduction

I sit beside the most frenetic river in the world - the Chao Phraya in Bangkok. Water taxis with V6 car engines attached to a stick propeller roar up and down, big boats, small boats, 10 million people and mega pollution, in order to consider an introduction to the benefits of meditation in yoga.

I am not a typical yoga person – someone who is a spiritual, flexible hippy, as Sarah Tucker's research has discovered.

I am a medical practitioner with twenty five years experience in helping people retain their youthfulness and making them look the best for their age. This involves prevention and intervention using professional skincare, skin rejuvenation procedures, fat reduction, Botox (r), dermal fillers, lasers, and in some cases the scalpel.

The ageing process is without question hastened with the stresses of everyday life and the big events - career change, divorce, bereavement and others. There are many instinctive and external coping mechanisms to help us manage these stresses. Tell the average sort of bloke that yoga might be of benefit and hear the cynical sniggering. When a trainer suggested yoga to me 10 years ago I choked on my espresso. It's not that I am now a yoga fanatic but the benefits I have found through a short weekly session are readily accessible to all.

Yoga can be totally physically exhausting, yes at the risk of repeating myself, absolutely knackering. I use a stretching routine which has greatly improved my posture and a back problem. Try holding a press up position and soon it becomes apparent you don't need any fancy gym equipment to work or stretch muscle.

Nor do you need, for risk of shooting myself in the foot, cosmetic surgery or the scalpel to look youthful. Find the right yoga teacher and you find a source of youth.

Sarah Tucker is the right yoga teacher. As Helen

Lederer comments, Sarah is a fun, empathetic, knowing spirit, and a born storyteller. It's appropriate she's also a novelist and travel writer because each yoga session is effectively a journey of self-discovery. You start stressed, you finish chilled. And you learn to breath properly.

We take our ability to breath for granted but when we think about breathing, suddenly we become aware of our ability to control the in- and exhalation which is scary. And it's an interesting contradiction that thinking about breathing whilst doing yoga brings a sense of relaxation, physical exertion and a mental emptying.

Stress makes us look older (check in the mirror after a late night). So any means of de-stressing, which yoga does, improves appearance, but only to a certain point.

The old saying "as a person thinks so they become" is true. If we feel good we look good, and if we look good we feel good about ourselves....a perfect circle! So take a deep breath, and regardless of what age, gender, shape or size you are, give yoga a go.

Dr Patrick Bowler, author of The Nervous Girls' Guide to Nip & Tuck, MS BS LRCP MRCS DRCOG

CHAPTER ONE

YOU CARRY YOUR EMOTIONAL BAGGAGE BADLY

We all have emotional baggage. Some of us just carry it better than others.

It would be odd if we didn't, behaving like some monolith that, whatever happens to us, reacts blank faced, like a Victoria Beckham to camera.

Life experience shapes our perception but we are more than the sum of our experiences because we grow and learn. Or we don't. We just make the same mistakes over and over again, until we take on the baggage as though it feels a part of us, or a piece of baggage we are holding onto. We then store it away, until the box bursts, frequently causing imbalances in our body. Sports and exercise psychologists identify that those most successful do not think about the past or future, but are completely focused on the 'now'. Anxiety impedes success and good self-esteem optimises progress. Yoga has been proven to reduce anxiety levels of those who practice regularly and improve levels of self-esteem. Of course, yoga alone does not rid you of emotional baggage, but the practice is an extremely effective tool if used with knowledge.

Yoga teaches us to listen to our body and what it is telling us about our wellbeing. Why does the left knee hurt and not the right? Why is there an ache in the right hip? These are the symptoms of emotional issues which lead to physical ones. The body is teaching us about our emotions; and how if we hold onto them, they are able to physically put us out of balance.

And it is nothing to do with how much other regular exercise we do. As a yoga instructor I get many runners and cyclists coming up to me asking about their knee. And it was always the left. The left knee in particular is connected with our fear and subconscious anxieties.

Something in their life had been going wrong, or not quite right, and they were worried about it, but trying to suppress their worries. But it came out, and their body told them something was out of balance.

We even use the word 'betrayed'. Our body 'betrayed' us. Our body language 'betrayed us', as though our body has let us down and done something dreadful. Our body has shown us, told us, helped us, guided us, to what is the issue. **Our bodies never lie to us. We should listen to our body more. We should listen to our emotions more. But what do we listen to? What is the one part of ourselves that we revere more than anything else? And leads us astray. Our mind. And what does our mind listen to? Other people's stuff.** So we are carrying other people's stuff. We are carrying not only our mind games, but their mind games as well. And unlike our emotions and our body, our mind lies to us. All the time. Few are able to tap into the subconscious, although you are able to through meditation.

And this is where yoga comes in.

Clear the mind. Take the mind out of the equation. Leave the mind, the thoughts at the door. And let the body and emotions take control in the yoga class. They work beautifully together. The body allows the emotions to express themselves. The emotions allow the body to be expressive. The body balances and releases the emotions. The emotions flood the body with energy. Hold your breath physically and you hold your breath emotionally. Just leave the mind at the door. In fact, it's not emotional baggage we carry badly, it's mind baggage.

YOGA – A BRIEF HISTORY

I held a survey of over five hundred people last year, ranging from eighteen year olds to eighty year olds around the UK, of their perception of yoga and asked for three words they would use to describe it. Some practiced yoga (about half), others did not. All ages, from professional sports people to teenagers who are stuck to their iPod, to OAPs. The words that came out the most were:

spiritual
flexible
hippy

So unless you are a flexible spiritual hippy, don't go anywhere near a yoga class.

True, it has become more mass market although some of the celebrities who practice appear a tad obsessive compulsive - although doubtless they would be even more so if they didn't practice yoga.

The yoga postures on the internet also show how bendy those who practice are, as though if you can't do a headstand, there's something wrong with you.

My perception of yoga was one of bendy bodies, looking emaciated and wearing 'barely there' clothes, with long flowing hair (the men and the women), people who treated yoga like a religion, praying at its altar in India, California, Thailand; anywhere they could lay their yoga mat, they would do a headstand. And everyone always looked so stern and so serious. As though they took not only their practice seriously but they took themselves seriously.

Those who practiced didn't seem happy. They didn't even look serene. They looked as though they were in need of a good meal and a good laugh. They looked as though they were in a bubble of their own making - and it wasn't one filled with bliss.

In the 1960s and 1970s yoga was almost exclusively the domain of the hippy movement and those who visited India, or Ibiza or anywhere that began with a vowel. If you hadn't visited India on some form of yoga retreat, preferably with a fast and a lot of joss sticks thrown in, you couldn't call yourself a yogi.

There was a woman on ITV who would appear for twenty minutes at seven o'clock on Sunday mornings, sitting on a backdrop of white, so white, she looked as though she was sitting on a cloud – or perhaps that was the illusion they wanted to create. She spoke in quiet, almost whisper-like tones about each pose and as a child I would watch her intently thinking 'how cool it was to be that cool', to bend her body, touch her toes, get her head up her backside in a back bend (later I learnt it was called 'camel pose', although I have never seen a camel do that) and at the end of half an hour look cool and serene and as though a piece of chocolate cake had never passed her lips to smudge her white pyjamas on the white backdrop. If it wasn't for her head, hands and feet showing, she would have almost disappeared.

In the eighties, it was all 'Jane Fonda Workout' and 'feel the burn' rather than chant the Omm. The antithesis of keeping still, it was high impact, bounce and stretch, hyper extend, and hyper extend again. I taught high impact aerobics in my twenties and now I think back to some of the movements we did in class – both as an instructor and a student – we must have caused so much damage unknowingly because at the time, that is how everyone trained – high impact.

In the nineties, we had Step class. Up down, up down, wonderful for the bottom, but hammered the knees. I remember going to a Step class on the date I was due to give birth to my son Tom, holding onto the bump with the instructor ready with a kettle just in case the waters broke. Yoga was just starting to make a resurgence towards the end of the nineties but it was still very much Step and kick boxing. Kicking the aggression out of the body. Anything to do with kicking, punching, jabbing was in. Yoga was out.

And then the noughties. People started to run marathons, half marathons, running machines, as gyms became more high tech with their equipment. And dance became fashionable again in all its forms – from ballroom, to modern, to jazz, tap, belly, anything Strictly Come Dancing could do, Zumba, Balletcize, and the dancers who first thought up aerobics came round again, but this time rather than doing the warm up for the dance (which is how aerobics started) they taught the dance itself.

All this running, jumping up and down (I've forgotten urban rebounding – little trampolines, wonderful cardio but lousy if you had bladder problems), kicking, punching, running, star jumping, did not deal with the fact at the end of a workout, our bodies felt good, the endorphins clicked in, but our minds were still racing, increasingly full of stuff we were filtering through, not just from the TV and newspapers, our friends and families, but also the internet and iPhones. We were being bombarded with unfiltered messages and were unable to filter it ourselves.

That's why I started yoga. Not because I needed to lengthen or strengthen my hamstrings or spine. Or be able to do a head or handstand. Nor because I wanted to somehow belong to an ethereal sect of people who could do such things. But I wanted to clear my mind of all the crap that had accumulated over the years. All the emotional baggage I was still carrying with me. About my divorce, the inadequacies I felt as a career woman, as a woman, as a mother, as a lover. As everything really. I had written about episodes in my life as novels. It was not a cathartic experience but more to understand why I had made the decisions I had. Like many others I had gone to counselling to understand how and why I had got myself into the situations I had. They made a good story. So good, I wrote several bestselling novels about them, which other people obviously identified with.

The Last Year of Being Single, and The Last Year of Being Married, The Younger Man, The Playground Mafia and The Control Freak Chronicles all tell the story about someone being manipulated and how she deals with it. The protagonist is someone who controls and intellectualises her emotions and lets her logic work things out - which is all very British (stiff upper lip) but lousy for the stress levels.

And yet it is the mind that got the protagonist (me) into the situation in the first place. The emotions are natural, normal, spontaneous, real. The reactions to them – the thought process in how I translate and act upon them – all comes from the mind.

Of course, I didn't learn these lessons by myself. I worked with clinical psychologists over the years for my novels, identifying how characters in the books would behave and should react. As a travel writer, I observed how different cultures behaved when things happened in their lives, such as bereavement, marriage, heartbreak, loneliness, and how cultures reacted differently. I realised how we are taught to observe and intellectualise our feelings rather than feel our feelings. We revere logic and the power of the mind, when it is the mind that causes us emotional and physical problems not the other way round. Yoga clears the mind and allows you to discipline it in the same way you do your body. And teaches you how to observe your body and learn from it. And that your emotions do not belong locked away in a box. They need to be expressed and listened to. This book shows you how.

WHY THIS BOOK?

There are many books out there about yoga, but none focus on specific emotional issues which yoga helps to alleviate. I observed over the years people coming to my classes and others who have arrived at the decision to start yoga not because they wanted to improve their flexibility but they wanted to improve their attitude towards life and themselves.

I took up yoga to deal with physical issues that were being caused by emotional imbalances and as a yoga instructor, I have observed that 100% of those I teach have physical issues which stem from emotional imbalances – not the other way round.

Yoga, more than anything else, helps you to express your emotions and find the calm again. The fact you will be more flexible, have a stronger core, have a positive disposition, be slower to anger, be able to think more clearly, feel and look younger is a by-product of a practice which isn't a cure all but is an essential part of the jigsaw puzzle to keeping a balance emotionally, mentally, physically and spiritually in your life.

Yoga makes you breath properly and be comfortable in your skin. It gives balance to your life, showing you how to get balance for yourself in everything you do. When all about you is chaos, it puts you in the eye of the storm so you are calm and stops you from being swept away by other people's stuff.

WHAT TYPE OF YOGA?

It's irrelevant. Of course you may have gone to a yoga class and thought it was not for you. This may be because you didn't click with the teacher or the type of yoga you chose. Yoga is as much psychological as it is physical. Remember you are dealing with the emotions and the body at the same time, so both need to be spoken to. So many instructors just focus on the physical, reciting sanskrit names of each asana perfectly but not explaining the purpose of each posture and why it works. Does it really matter if I am able to touch my toes? Will it make me a bad person if I don't breath through my abdominals? I didn't get the point of yoga until I took a trip to India. I didn't even go for the yoga. I went to observe the tigers with my son.

My last stop was in Delhi. We stayed at a modern hotel which offered a crack of dawn morning yoga session. My son (thirteen at the time) was not interested. I was, and although the room was small, off a modern gym, not situated in a fragrant garden or with incense filling the air and soothing music in the background or any of the other accessories that accompany classes, the instructor (who was smiling, and looked nothing like the solemn, flexible spiritual hippy I had anticipated) explained to me why the breath is important. He explained why yoga was relevant to my life or any life. He explained why I should breath from the abdominals and not the chest. How it calms the breath, calms the spirit, how yoga turns anxiety to excitement and how you don't have to hyper ventilate to have fun.

I laughed in his yoga class. I had never seen anyone smile in a yoga class, let alone laugh. I didn't think it was allowed. I understood for the first time how yoga is good for the soul and the identity and the emotional balance, because in that modern hotel, in that busy city, in that modern gym, I realised why the emotional benefits of yoga probably surpass those of the physical because they are interconnected.

I returned home, beginning to understand its full potential and started to investigate the different types of yoga. Iyengar (precision and detail), flow (one movement into the next), power (Americanised feel the burn exercise called yoga), Hatha (about the breath) and ashtanga (competitive). I chose to go with the flow. It suited me as it seemed the most dance-like and rhythmic. I also enjoyed Iyengar, with its precision; I recognised the discipline I had experienced when learning dance – the importance of posture, of detail and I felt it was useful to try out different types of yoga, because they all had their benefits. Even hot yoga or Bikram, where you have a range of movements in a very hot studio, is excellent for strengthening your breath in particular. If you could calm your breath and learn to breath through your nose in ninety degree heat, you could do it anywhere.

WHO IS THE BOOK FOR?

The A To Zen Of Yoga focuses on how specific yoga asanas and sequences rid you of emotional baggage and how they can be done anywhere. At the airport, waiting for the bus, even sitting on the bus, on the train, and in your own home. You don't need a white light backdrop, you don't need to be emaciated or have gone to an expensive yoga retreat in Sri Lanka, nor do you need the full yoga gear.

Breath and alignment are important. Having a sense of mischief and the ridiculous is useful. Yoga is a meditation with movement. Meditation is not just the cross legged posture at the beginning and at the end of the practice. And you don't have to do an hour and a half yoga class daily. If all you can fit in is five minutes, five minutes will do. When you breath, align your body and close your mind, you are in a state of meditation in each posture. When I teach now I often ask the class to close their eyes during parts of the yoga practice (although I don't want them to fall over and crack their head open in the process) and realise how much their breath slows and deepens, how their alignment improves and how their sense of self judgement disappears. They literally 'see' with better eyes when their eyes are closed.

The A to Zen of Yoga shows how yoga helps you in everyday life. How anyone can do it, whatever age, size, shape or gender. I instruct rugby players, rowers, skiers, cyclists, all at professional level, all extremely focussed, highly competitive, but all of whom have issues which destabilise their focus. And they never stretch enough.

I have studied sports psychology to understand more about body dysmorphia, a growing trend in all ages, not just the young. Obsessive compulsives even obsess about yoga, which is ironic because yoga is about balance, so I have chosen postures in this book which help with obsessive compulsive behaviour - even if it results in doing less yoga. It's all about quality not quantity.

The A to Zen of Yoga will show you not only why certain postures are good for ridding yourself of emotional baggage but why this happens. It shows you the potential errors you could make – which could do more harm than good. I will mention the sanskrit because the language is beautiful and over time you will think so too, but don't feel you have to learn it by rote and if you can't name the posture, you can't do the posture. That's rubbish. So let go of your stuff, don't take on anyone else's and go with the flow.

CHAPTER TWO

HOW TO CARRY YOUR EMOTIONS

Anxious, depressed, lonely, heartbroken, tired, lacking in focus, self-absorbed, angry, jealous, envious, greedy, vain, impatient, vengeful? Or all of the above?

Stand back from the emotion and look at it as though it doesn't belong to you. As though you have the feeling in your hand and want to study it rather than feel it. Take this 'feeling' with you as you practice and allow the body to feel it and release it. Let it go. Breath it in then breath it out. Accept it and let it go. You will feel lighter and more balanced and energetic and this will show in your postures, your work-life balance, even your eyes, hair and skin.

IF A THOUGHT COMES INTO YOUR MIND...

If a thought comes into your mind, observe it don't judge it. Don't fight it, as you will think of it more. If I told you to not think about a tomato, you would think about a tomato. If I made it imperative to not think about a tomato - for example, give a punishment - you would think about it even more. Or lie to me. Treat your thoughts like pebbles. Pick it up, observe it and throw it in a lake. Let it go. There will be some thoughts, memories that will be heavier than others. More difficult to let go of. They may appear small, but when you pick them up they are heavy. They weigh heavy on you and keep you out of balance. For example like a past relationship that chips away at your confidence.

Or the thoughts may be large; like huge boulders rather than pebbles, but when you pick them up to throw them into the lake, they are as light as a feather. Issues which appear large are in fact easier to get rid of than those niggling ones that insist on coming back when you least expect.

If for example it's cold in the studio, you feel cold, when was the last time you felt cold, in your home this morning, when you couldn't find your purse, have you lost it, should you go to the police?....... Throw it in the lake. The thought that is, not the purse.

Over five years I asked many yogis what makes them happy. Yoga is not the tonic to cure all evils, but it is one of them. These are the others...

Here's ten things happy people don't care for.

1. AGE

Indeed, age is just a number. And happy people know this.

They don't let this ever-increasing number define who they are and what they do. They just do whatever it is they want!

2. CARING ABOUT WHAT OTHERS THINK OR SAY

This is one of the biggest blocks to our happiness.

Happy people don't care for that. They recognise that the words of others are never accurate and should never judge them for who they are and what they're capable of.

3. JOBS

That's not to say happy people are unemployed.

The key idea is: You're not your job.

What matters more is your talent, passion and outlook on life. Allowing your job to take over any of that would only mean you're allowing a label to define who you are.

4. FEAR

Fear is not real. Happy people know that.

With that, they know that the nervousness and anxiety that supposedly comes with fear are not real. They block it out, get out of their comfort zone, feel a little crazy and just do what they want anyway.

There's just no point holding back in life just because you feel a little scared.

5. THE NEGATIVE STATE OF THE WORLD

There's a lot of disturbing stuff going on out there. War, protests, riots, animals going extinct or innocent people having bad things happen to them.

Happy people don't deny any of these, but they do a good job in making sure it doesn't affect how they feel.

The happiest people I know simply focus on trying to make the world a better place, one small step at a time. They may not be able to start a revolution overnight, but they know that by showing a little kindness and compassion to our fellow man, the world is that much more positive already. Don't let the negative in life get to you. It's not your fault others have made it this way.

6. TOXIC PEOPLE

"You're the average of the five people you spend the most time with".

Ever had to deal with an annoying friend or somebody who's just really self-destructive?

Dump them. It's time to create a positive environment for yourself.

Happy people gain happiness from the people they are with and not just from within. If you're feeling unhappy, take a look around. Sometimes it's the people that are just dragging you down.

7. THE PAST OR THE FUTURE

The past does not exist, neither does the future.

If you want to be happy, you've got to let go of the past and move on with life. Learn from it and grow from it, then make sure you don't repeat the same mistakes.

As for the future, happy people pretty much let go of expectations.

When you let go of the past and future, then you can truly enjoy the present.

8. EXPECTING ANYTHING IN RETURN

Start doing things for the sake of doing things. Help others for the sake of being compassionate. The true reward is knowing that you've added positivity to others.

Happy people let go of always wanting something in return. That's how they never get disappointed.

9. COMPLAINING

Complaining is the result of an unhappy life. Sometimes things don't go your way. You can't escape that.

Happy people know that. They're grateful for what they have instead and then they try to find the solution with a positive mindset.

10. CONFORMING TO SOCIETY'S STANDARDS

Just like age, there are a lot of labels out there that try to define who we are. Expectations are always thrown at us and it can be pretty overwhelming at times.

Happy people don't care for any of that. They look within and do what they want in life.

This is how happiness is created. Not doing things you don't care for.

CHAPTER THREE

WHICH POSTURES WORK

So now you know how to observe your emotions and go with them, how to treat your thoughts like pebbles and not fight or judge them just let them go, and how to be happy? (or how other people maintain 'happy') here are the postures/asanas which focus on specific emotional issues.

I'm not suggesting you do a back bend in the middle of the board room or a hand stand in the middle of a restaurant or dance floor. But taking time out in the morning and evening to do specific yoga practice or ideally joining a class and speaking to your instructor, is an excellent way to deal with emotional issues.

Counselling is about 'talking' - analysing and intellectualising feelings, so the brain and intellect becomes engaged again - finding cause for how we feel but not actually allowing us to experience the feeling. We want to get rid of the anger, the loneliness, the grief, the lack of focus, the jealousy, but before we do, we need to accept it and show ourselves compassion. That is what our body is telling us when we store the emotion. We need to observe it, recognise it is there and then let it go. As a culture we are not good at doing this. We box in and suppress emotion until it bursts.

Yoga teaches us to observe ourselves rather than judge ourselves. The difference between judging ourselves and observing ourselves is acceptance and compassion. When we observe, we are open to learning, we let go of stuff, we create space in our mind and heart and body for positives. When we judge, we close down, we create limitations on ourselves, we restrict ourselves, we hold onto stuff. Listen to your breath when you are judging yourself or someone else - you will realise it becomes quicker, tighter and you actually become short of breath. When you are observing, your breath becomes stronger, deeper, longer. Observe, don't judge.

What we need to do is 'feel the feelings', stop putting them into little boxes because they are inconvenient and make us anti-social. We should stop intellectualising our emotions - and start accepting them. As someone who has written numerous 'relationship' books on how to deal with emotional issues, its' only when I started yoga, I realised it was feeling them that would enable me to release my emotions - not analysing them.

One last thing. **In the film Forest Gump, there is a scene when he is standing over the grave of his wife 'Jenny' and speaking very eloquently about how he will look after their son; how it was for the best because she was in a lot of pain; how he knows she is in heaven and that is what he tells himself and his son every day. That she knows she was loved and that their son will be safe. And then he is quiet for a few moments. And says 'then why does it still hurt so much?'**

The head can rationalise as much as it likes. If you don't take your heart with you on your journey, you go nowhere.

ANGER MANAGEMENT

Yoga can help you to relax and de-stress. Don't repress it, allow yourself to experience emotion. But instead of reacting in destructive ways, channel energy.

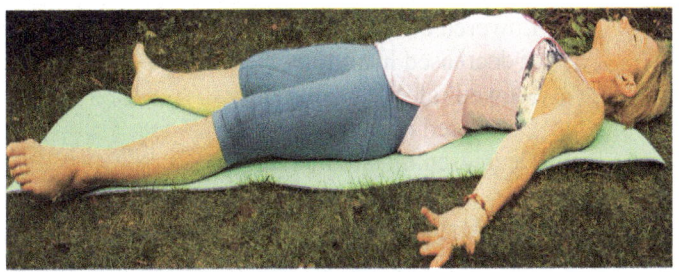

CORPSE POSE OR SAVASANA

Quietens your mind and stills your body. Lie flat on your back with your legs close but not touching and your arms parallel to the body, with the palms facing up. Close your eyes, relax your facial muscles and breath deeply and slowly through the nostrils. Focus on consciously relaxing each part of your body, starting with your head and working your way down. If you begin to feel sleepy, breath more quickly and deeply.

SPECIAL NOTE ON SAVASANA

Though it's sometimes used to begin practice, Savasana is most often used to end practice, to allow your body, mind, and spirit to fully relax and release tension. It's a time to let lingering thoughts and worries fade away. From the depth and darkness of Savasana, you can be rejuvenated, refreshed, and reborn.

The deeply relaxing aspect of Savasana is known to be therapeutic for stress. When you're under stress, your sympathetic nervous system produces a "fight or flight" response that can over-stimulate your mind and body, causing anxiety, fatigue, depression, and disease. Conversely, practicing Savasana stimulates the parasympathetic nervous system — known as the "rest and digest" response. Relaxing the physical body in Savasana has numerous benefits, including:

> Lowered blood pressure
> A decreased heart rate
> Slowed rate of respiration
> Decreased muscle tension
> Decreased metabolic rate

The physical response can further result in:

> Reduced occurrence of headaches
> Relief from fatigue and insomnia
> Reduced nervous tension
> Relief from anxiety and panic attacks
> Increased overall energy levels
> Increased productivity
> Improved concentration and memory
> Clear-headedness and a sense of focus
> Heightened self-confidence

In addition to the mind-body benefits, Savasana is also a time during your practice when you can connect with your peaceful, innermost self. The word "yoga" is often translated as "union," referring to the connection between your mind, body, and spirit. When you settle into Savasana and become aware of this connection, you are truly practicing yoga.

Savasana is appropriate for all yoga students. If you are uncomfortable lying on your back, practice a supported version of the pose. Women who are pregnant should keep their head and chest raised in the pose by resting on a bolster or cushion. Always work within your own range of limits and abilities. If you have any medical concerns, talk with your doctor before practicing yoga.

STEP BY STEP

Lie on your back with your legs straight and arms at your sides. Rest your hands about six inches away from your body with your palms up. Let your feet drop open. Close your eyes. You may want to cover your body with a blanket.

Let your breath occur naturally.

Allow your body to feel heavy on the ground.

Working from the soles of your feet up to the crown of your head, consciously release every body part, organ, and cell.

Relax your face. Let your eyes drop deep into their sockets. Invite peace and silence into your mind, body, and soul.

Stay in Savasana for five minutes for every 30 minutes of your practice.

To exit the pose, first begin to deepen your breath. Bring gentle movement and awareness back to your body, wiggling your fingers and toes. Roll to your right side and rest there for a moment. With an inhalation, gently press yourself into a comfortable seated position.

Let your head be the last thing to come into place. Carry the peace and stillness of Savasana with you throughout the rest of your day.

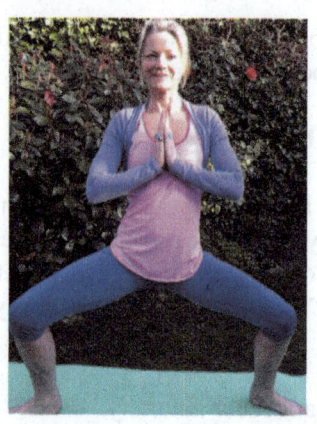

GODDESS POSE: UTKATA KONASANA

Do not practice this pose if you have a recent or chronic injury to the legs, hips, back, or shoulders. Always work within your own range of limits and abilities. If you have any medical concerns, talk with your doctor before practicing yoga.

STEP BY STEP

Begin standing in Mountain Pose (Tadasana) at the top of your mat with your arms at your sides. Bring your hands to rest comfortably on your hips.
Turn to the right and step your feet wide apart, about four feet.

Turn your toes out slightly, so they point to the corners of your mat.

On an exhalation, bend your knees directly over your toes and lower your hips into a squat. Work toward bringing your thighs parallel to the floor, but do not force yourself into the squat.

Extend your arms out to the sides at shoulder-height with your palms facing down. Then, spiral your thumbs up toward the ceiling, so your palms face forward. Bend your elbows and point your fingertips toward the ceiling; your upper arms and forearms should be at a 90 degree angle.

Tuck your tailbone in slightly and press your hips forward as you draw your thighs back. Keep your knees in line with your toes. Soften your shoulders. Gaze softly at the horizon.

Hold for up to ten breaths. To release, slowly return your hands to your hips. Keeping your spine upright, inhale as you press firmly into your feet and straighten your legs. Step your feet together and come back to the top of your mat in Mountain Pose.

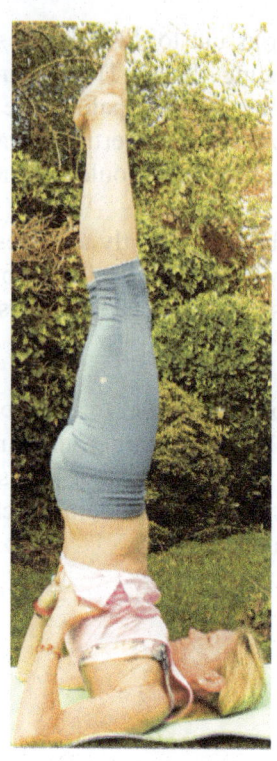

SHOULDER STAND OR SARVANGASANA

The shoulder stand reduces excessive anger and hate, as well as invigorating your body. Don't perform this if you have breathing difficulties, neck problems or upper back pain.

STEP BY STEP

Begin in a seated position with legs extended long and together and arms relaxed on either side. Take a big inhalation. On the exhalation, fall forward, pulling navel to spine and extending hands toward feet as much or as little as feels good on the legs and lower back. Allow head to relax down toward legs. (If hamstrings are tight, soften knees.) Breath here for as long as it feels good.

When you are ready to come out, one vertebra at a time, roll up and then onto your back, keeping soft knees. Bend knees and place feet on the floor with arms on either side. Soften knees and press arms into the ground to reach feet up toward the ceiling. Breath here for as long as is comfortable.

When you feel comfortable, allow feet to fall back behind you an amount that feels good on your neck.

Reach feet to the ground for plough pose. Clasp hands together on the ground and wiggle shoulders underneath you one at a time. Press firmly into arms, reach through heels, and breath here for at least three deep breaths.

From plough or modified plough, place hands on lower back for support and try to keep elbows about shoulder-width apart. Soften legs and allow knees to rest on forehead. Breath here for as long as is comfortable.

When you feel steady, reach feet toward the ceiling one at a time, lengthening legs when you feel comfortable. Breath here for at least three deep breaths. To come down, slowly soften knees toward forehead, come back to plough, and slowly lower back to mat one vertebra at a time.

Fish pose is a great counterpart to shoulder stand and can be an effective way to relieve neck and back pain, improve circulation, and open your chest muscles.

Place hands and palms underneath butt and hips. Keep elbows as close together as possible and fingertips facing forward with forearms parallel to each other on the ground. Bend elbows and lean onto forearms, pressing them into the floor. Lift chest up toward the ceiling so that back is arched. Bring elbows toward each other until they're about shoulder-width apart. Allow head to relax down toward the ground until it touches the mat. Breath here for at least three deep breaths. When ready, come out of this slowly and lie on your back for a few breaths to enjoy how great you feel.

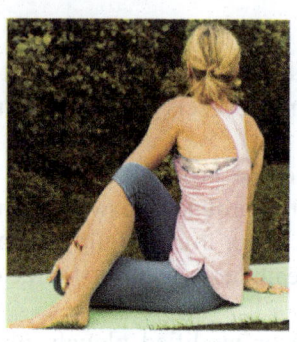

HALF TWIST POSE OR ARDHA MATSYENDRASANA

When our lower bodies act as foundation for the upper body to spiral around in a twist, transformative changes bless our inner organs. Specifically the liver and the spleen benefit from the Half Spinal Twist as we inhale fresh, new life, and allow all that is old and stale to be washed away.

The liver, according to Chinese medicine, is where the majority of our anger resides in the body. We create toxins in this vital organ when we hold on to hurts, grudges, and resentments. With each inhalation, lengthen the spine and invite the Prana of the breath to bathe the liver. Consider a relationship, either with yourself or another, where you are holding on to the hot fire of anger. On the cooling exhalation, spiral your belly, rib cage, and upper chest around to the back. Go beyond surface level as you deepen into the grace of understanding, beginning to release all the anger you have stored up that no longer serves you. Choose compassion as you transform anger into forgiveness. Breath by breath, relax deeper into the twist, opening up space inside you for greater joy.

STEP BY STEP

Sit on the floor with your legs straight out in front of you, buttocks supported on a folded blanket. Bend your knees, put your feet on the floor, then slide your left foot under your right leg to the outside of your right hip. Lay the outside of the left leg on the floor. Step the right foot over the left leg and stand it on the floor outside your left hip. The right knee will point directly up at the ceiling.

Exhale and twist toward the inside of the right thigh. Press the right hand against the floor just behind your right buttock, and set your left upper arm on the outside of your right thigh near the knee. Pull your front torso and inner right thigh snugly together.

Press the inner right foot very actively into the floor, release the right groin, and lengthen the front torso. Lean the upper torso back slightly, against the shoulder blades, and continue to lengthen the tailbone into the floor.

You can turn your head in one of two directions: continue the twist of the torso by turning it to the right, or counter the twist of the torso by turning it left and looking over the left shoulder at the right foot.

With every inhalation, lift a little more through the sternum, pushing the fingers against the floor to help. Twist a little more with every exhalation. Be sure to distribute the twist evenly throughout the entire length of the spine; don't concentrate it in the lower back.

Stay for 30 seconds to one minute, then release with an exhalation, return to the starting position, and repeat to the left for the same length of time.

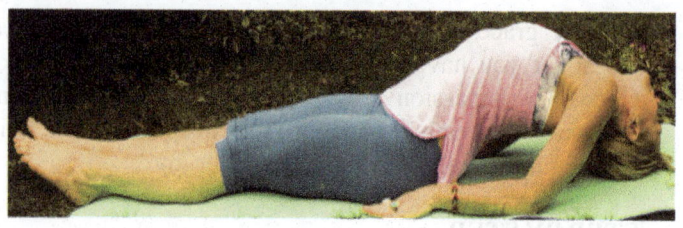

FISH POSE OR MATSYASANA

This particular posture is usually practiced following the Shoulder Stand as a counter-balance. After turning your world upside down, it's now time to focus on expanding and opening the heart and lung area. Fear often settles in this area, creating a kind of static that keeps us from being able to clearly hear our loving inner voice.

As your body weight rests on your legs, buttocks, forearms and the crown of the head, lift the rib cage and upper chest area as high as it will go upward. Create an opening directly from your heart...

STEP BY STEP

Lie on your back on the floor with your knees bent, feet on the floor. Inhale, lift your pelvis slightly off the floor, and slide your hands, palms down, below your buttocks. Then rest your buttocks on the backs of your hands (and don't lift them off your hands as you perform this pose). Be sure to tuck your forearms and elbows up close to the sides of your torso.

Inhale and press your forearms and elbows firmly against the floor.

Next press your scapulas into your back and, with an inhalation, lift your upper torso and head away from the floor.

Then release your head back onto the floor. Depending on how high you arch your back and lift your chest, either the back of your head or its crown will rest on the floor.

There should be a minimal amount of weight on your head to avoid crunching your neck.

You can keep your knees bent or straighten your legs out onto the floor. If you do the latter, keep your thighs active, and press out through the heels.

Stay for 15 to 30 seconds, breathing smoothly. With an exhalation, lower your torso and head to the floor. Draw your thighs up into your belly and squeeze.

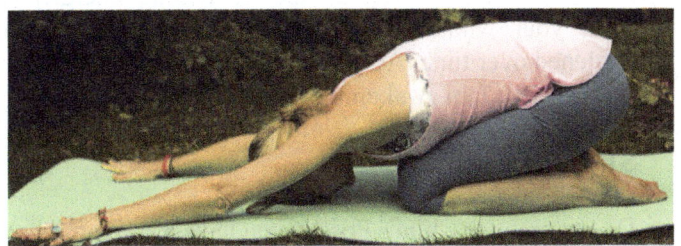

CHILD POSE OR BALASANA

One of the main resting poses of yoga practice, child's pose involves sitting on the knees and bending forward with arms forward or by your side. It is comforting and self-soothing. It slows the mind and helps us focus on the breath. This asana gently stretches your lower back, hips, thighs, knees, and ankles, relaxes your spine, shoulders and neck, increases blood circulation to your head (which reduces headaches), massages your internal organs and calms the mind (central nervous system), thus helping relieve stress and tension.

With the innocence and unselfconsciousness of a small child, rest your upper body along your upper thighs as your hips melt down toward your heels. Allow your forehead to find its support on the Earth as you feel nurtured and protected at the same time. In this safe space, with your eyes closed and your gaze internally focused, become aware of the grief pangs which are residing in your heart.

Who has passed from your life? Which relationship have you lost? What sadness remains?

As you breath deeply into your child body, let your heart open the door into your emotional field and observe what lies within you. The child is faithful in each moment to whatever emotion is awake and alive. Be the child, feeling fully and not holding anything back.

Cry if the tears come streaming down.

Let memories of that which has passed flood your being. Mother yourself in the nourishing energies that relax your whole being and soften the grief that has hardened over time. As the river of grief is liberated, feel a sense of freedom awakening inside you.

STEP BY STEP

Do not practice Child's Pose if you have a current or recent knee injury. Women who are pregnant should only practice a wide-legged variation of the pose — do not press the belly on top of the thighs. Always work within your own range of limits and abilities. If you have any medical concerns, talk with your doctor before practicing yoga.

Begin on your hands and knees. Centre your breath, and begin to let your thoughts slow down. Turn your awareness inward.

Spread your knees wide apart while keeping your big toes touching. Rest your buttocks on your heels.

Those with very tight hips can keep their knees and thighs together.

Sit up straight and lengthen your spine up through the crown of your head.

On an exhalation, bow forward, draping your torso between your thighs. Your heart and chest should rest between or on top of your thighs. Allow your forehead to come to the floor.

Keep your arms long and extended, palms facing down. Press back slightly with your hands to keep your buttocks in contact with your heels. Lengthen from your hips to your armpits, and then extend even further through your fingertips.

For deeper relaxation, bring your arms back to rest alongside your thighs with your palms facing up. Completely relax your elbows.

Let your upper back broaden. Soften and relax your lower back. Allow all tension in your shoulders, arms, and neck to drain away.

Keep your gaze drawn inward with your eyes closed.

Hold for up to a minute or longer, breathing softly.

To release the pose, gently use your hands to walk your torso upright to sit back on your heels.

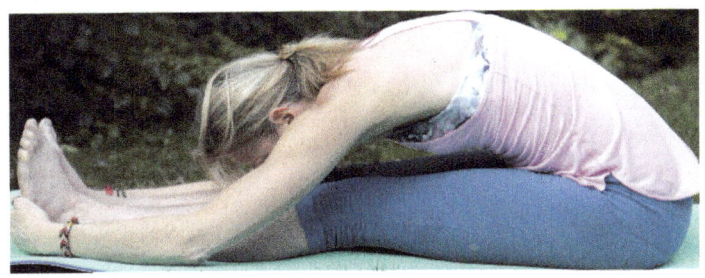

SEATED FORWARD BEND OR PASCHIMOTTANASANA

Beginning in the staff pose, raise arms up to the sky, and then bow your upper body down over your upper legs. Our hands rest softly on our legs or feet, wherever they can reach, and little by little the central channel of the spine gives way to the sweet pull of gravity. In forward bends, we invite a calming of the mind – the monkey mind with all of its worries and frets, its many variations of 'what ifs'.

Just for this moment, be completely present. The future lies far away from the next inhalation and exhalation, and it is not yours to fret over or attempt to control. Trust your strong legs, now connected to the ground beneath them, to support you in letting go fully with your upper body. Surrender the worries clouding your sky mind, allow yourself to go deeper into the physical fold, and open up to the vast expanse of peace that has been waiting patiently to bless you.

LACKING FOCUS

Is your mind racing in all directions and unable to focus on any one thing? You may be at rest but your mind never is. You are exhausted when you wake up, having run a marathon mentally in your sleep. How do you still the mind so you improve concentration?

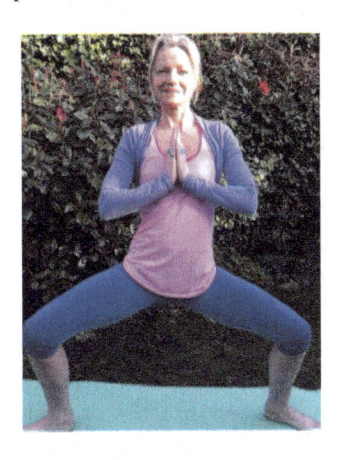

GODDESS POSE OR UTKATA KONASANA

Stretching your hips groin and chest, this posture strengthens and tones your core muscles, your quadriceps and inner thigh muscles, your shoulders, arms and upper back, heats the body and increases circulation.

STEP BY STEP

Do not practice this pose if you have had a recent or chronic injury to the legs, hips, back, or shoulders. Always work within your own range of limits and abilities. If you have any medical concerns, talk with your doctor before practicing yoga.

Begin standing in Mountain Pose (Tadasana) at the top of your mat with your arms at your sides. Bring your hands to rest comfortably on your hips.

Turn to the right and step your feet wide apart, about four feet. Turn your toes out slightly, so they point to the corners of your mat.

On an exhalation, bend your knees directly over your toes and lower your hips into a squat. Work toward bringing your thighs parallel to the floor, but do not force yourself into the squat.

Extend your arms out to the sides at shoulder-height with your palms facing down. Then, spiral your thumbs up toward the ceiling, so your palms face forward. Bend your elbows and point your fingertips toward the ceiling; your upper arms and forearms should be at a 90 degree angle.

Tuck your tailbone in slightly and press your hips forward as you draw your thighs back. Keep your knees in line with your toes. Soften your shoulders. Gaze softly at the horizon.

Hold for up to ten breaths. To release, slowly return your hands to your hips. Keeping your spine upright, inhale as you press firmly into your feet and straighten your legs. Step your feet together and come back to the top of your mat in Mountain Pose.

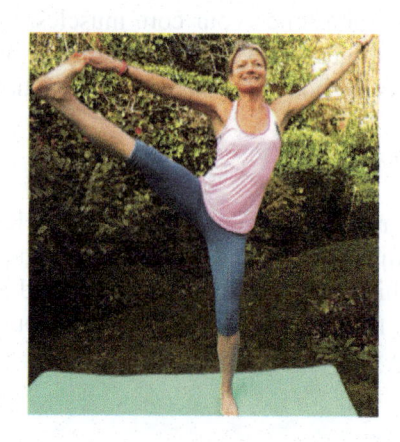

EXTENDED HAND TO TOE POSE OR UTTIHITA HASTA PADANGUSTHASANA

Stretching hamstrings and hips, this asana strengthens the back and arm muscles, improves sense of balance and calms the mind, which in turn improves focus.

STEP BY STEP

From Tadasana, bring your left knee toward your belly. Reach your left arm inside the thigh, cross it over the front ankle, and hold the outside of your left foot. If your hamstrings are tight, hold a strap looped around the left sole.

Firm the front thigh muscles of the standing leg, and press the outer thigh inward.

Inhale and extend the left leg forward. Straighten the knee as much as possible. If you're steady, swing the leg out to the side. Breath steadily; breathing takes concentration, but it helps you balance.

Hold for 30 seconds, then swing the leg back to centre with an inhalation, and lower the foot to the floor with an exhalation. Repeat on the other side for the same length of time.

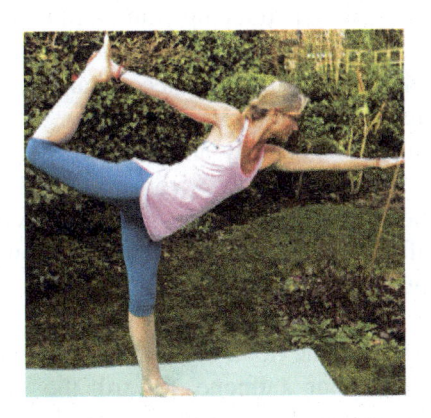

LORD OF THE DANCE POSE OR NATARASJASANA

Develops concentration and balance, tones and stretches the leg and hip muscles and develops range of motion in the shoulders. This asana also expands the chest and front body and strengthens the back body in a back bend.

STEP BY STEP

Do not practice this pose if you have a recent or chronic ankle or lower back injury. Also avoid this pose if you are currently experiencing low blood pressure, dizziness, migraines, or insomnia. Always work within your own range of limits and abilities. If you have any medical concerns, talk with your doctor before practicing yoga.

Begin standing in Mountain Pose (Tadasana) with your feet together and your arms at your sides.

Shift your weight onto your left foot.

Bend your right knee and bring your right heel toward your right buttock. Reach your right hand down and clasp your right foot's inner ankle. You can also loop a strap around the top of your right foot, and then hold onto the strap with your right hand. Draw your knees together.

Reach your left arm overhead, pointing your fingertips toward the ceiling and facing your palm to the right.

Fix your gaze softly at an unmoving spot in front of you. Make sure your left kneecap and toes continue to point directly forward.

When you feel steady and comfortable, begin to press your right foot away from your body as you simultaneously lean your torso slightly forward. Keep your chest lifting and continue reaching your left hand's fingertips up toward the ceiling.

Raise your right foot as high as you can. Bring your left thigh parallel to the floor, or higher if possible. At the same time, press your tailbone toward the floor to avoid compressing your lower back. Do not let your right knee splay open to the side.

If you are comfortable and steady here, you may go into the advanced pose. Swivel your right elbow forward and then up, so it points toward the ceiling. You will need to drop your right shoulder slightly as you make this adjustment. Hug your right bicep toward your right ear. Your right forearm should now be reaching overhead and behind your body to hold onto your foot or the strap. Bend your left elbow and reach your left hand back to hold onto your foot or the strap. Draw both arms inward toward your head as you keep your shoulder blades pressing down your back.

As you press your raised foot back, keep your chest lifting. Do not let your torso drop forward. Keep your pelvis square and your right knee drawn in toward the midline of your body.

If you are holding a strap, walk your hands down the strap toward your foot until you can clasp the top of your foot with both hands.

Hold for five breaths. To release, very slowly and gently return to your starting position. Then lower your right foot and come back into Mountain Pose. Repeat the pose on the opposite side for the same amount of time.

TIREDNESS

I'm not talking physically tired – but emotionally tired, where you can't think straight as there is so much going on in your head. It is exhausting, all that stuff we keep up in our heads. A combination of what we need to do today, should have done yesterday and need to do tomorrow or the week after.

Emotional fatigue has an impact on the physical. The more most of us do, the more we are able to do, the less we do, the less we are able to do, because our minds become bogged down with petty issues which when we have something constructive to focus on, we have no time for.

Helping to focus the mind and clear it from all the 'stuff' is the best way to alleviate tiredness. Tiredness is also caused by lack of proper sleep and yoga is excellent for insomnia. These postures in particular are good for both improving focus and for insomnia.

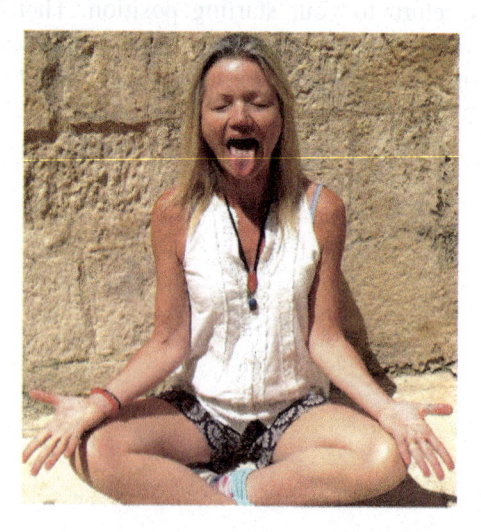

LION POSE OR SIMHASANA

Similar to the roar of the lion, this asana is performed in the exact fashion to draw as much usefulness as possible. The asana depicts the fierceness of the lion, which benefits those parts of the body where it is stretched and pulled.

This asana is very different to other asanas as it benefits your face, which many of the asanas are not able to do. It benefits your face, jaw, mouth, throat and tongue. If you have sore throat problems, this asana proves to be very useful.

Problems like tightness of the jaw, teeth grinding and clenched jaws can get some relief by performing this asana regularly. It involves the stretching of the tongue, as you are required to mimic the roaring lion. It can be treated as a very good asana which can remove your wrinkles and can be described as anti-ageing. We pay lot of attention to the other parts of our body and hardly take care of our face while performing the yoga asanas.

This asana may prove to be the most important asana you ever do. The muscles and tissues of your face have restored their lost charm to make your face more radiant than ever. It makes your face a beaming glory by performing this asana. The stretching and pulling stimulates the nerves to give you a refreshed look.

The blood circulation in the face also improves, thereby improving the circulation of oxygen and nutrients to the face. The gaze which is used in the asana helps your eyes by keeping them shiny and bright. It removes the tension from the eyes and also clears burning sensations which you keep feeling in your eyes.

The Lion Pose provides good stimulation to the nerves in the eyes and therefore helps in correcting weaknesses in vision. People suffering from respiratory ailments such as asthma and bronchitis can also benefit from practicing the Lion Pose regularly. Furthermore, neck and back pain can also be treated with the Lion Pose.

Compared to other conventional medications and drugs, there are no side effects which can negatively affect one's health. Alternative practices like yoga are always considered a safer option compared to traditional medical methods and procedures.

STEP BY STEP

Kneel on the floor and cross the front of the right ankle over the back of the left. The feet will point out to the sides. Sit back so the perineum snuggles down onto the top (right) heel. Press your palms firmly against your knees. Fan the palms and splay your fingers like the sharpened claws of a large feline.

Take a deep inhalation through the nose. Then simultaneously open your mouth wide and stretch your tongue out, curling its tip down toward the chin, open your eyes wide, contract the muscles on the front of your throat, and exhale the breath slowly out through your mouth with a distinct "ha" sound. The breath should pass over the back of the throat. You can roar two or three times. Then change the cross of the legs and repeat for the same number of times.

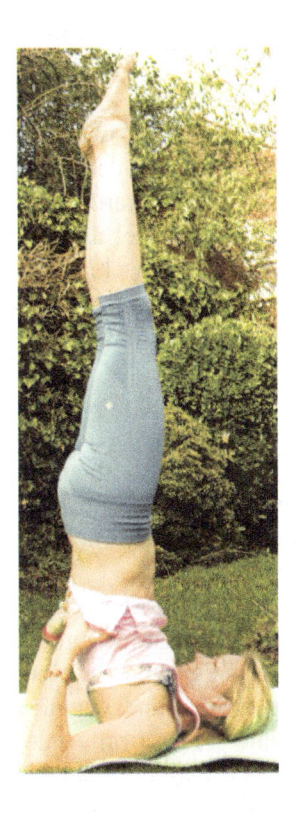

SUPPORTED SHOULDER STAND OR SALAMBA SARVANGASANA

Inversions help you get out of the 'monkey mind' by putting you in a different position to normal life. They literally turn things upside down, and stress and anxiety are a perception of danger and unease, and when you can get out of your mind – that helps. This posture tones your legs, buttocks, back and core muscles, stretches your shoulders and improves the flexibility of your upper spine.

It also calms the brain and nervous system, therefore helping to relieve stress, improves digestion and massages and stimulates the thyroid and prostate glands and flushes mucous from your lungs.

STEP BY STEP

Begin in a seated position with legs extended long and together and arms relaxed on either side. Take a big inhale. On the exhalation, fall forward, pulling navel to spine and extending hands toward feet as much or as little as feels good on legs and lower back. Allow your head to relax down toward your legs. (If hamstrings are tight, soften knees.) Breath here for as long as it feels good.

When you are ready to come out, one vertebra at a time, roll up and then onto back, keeping soft knees. Bend knees and place feet on the floor with arms on either side. Soften knees and press arms into the ground to reach feet up toward the ceiling. Breath here for as long as it is comfortable.

When you feel comfortable, allow feet to fall back behind you an amount that feels good on your neck.

Reach feet to the ground for plough pose. Clasp hands together on the ground and wiggle shoulders underneath you one at a time. Press firmly into arms, reach through heels, and breath here for at least three deep breaths.

From plough or modified plough, place hands on lower back for support and try to keep elbows about shoulder-width apart. Soften legs and allow knees to rest on forehead. Breath here for as long as it is comfortable.

When you feel steady, reach your feet toward the ceiling one at a time, lengthening legs when you feel comfortable. Breath here for at least three deep breaths. To come down, slowly soften knees toward forehead, come back to plough, and slowly lower back to mat one vertebra at a time.

Fish pose is a great counterpart to shoulder stand and can be an effective way to relieve neck and back pain, improve circulation, and open your chest muscles.

Place hands and palms underneath butt and hips. Keep elbows as close together as possible and fingertips facing forward with forearms parallel to each other on the ground. Bend elbows and lean onto forearms, pressing them into the floor.

Lift chest up toward the ceiling so that back is arched. Bring elbows toward each other until they're about shoulder-width apart.

Allow head to relax down toward the ground until it touches the mat. Breath here for at least three deep breaths. When ready, come out of this slowly and lie on your back for a few breaths to enjoy how great you feel.

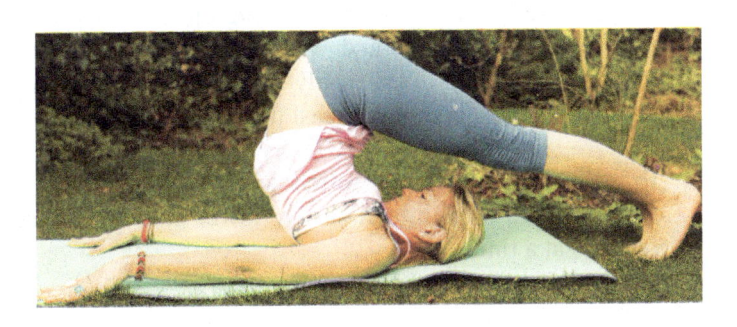

PLOUGH POSE OR HALASANA

This posture stretches the shoulders and improves the flexibility of your spine, calms your brain and nervous system and helps relieve stress and fatigue, improves digestion, massages and stimulates the thyroid gland, massages the abdominal organs and improves digestion, helps relieve the symptoms of menopause, and flushes mucous from your lungs.

STEP BY STEP

Begin in a seated position with legs extended long and together and arms relaxed on either side. Take a big inhalation. On the exhalation, fall forward, pulling navel to spine and extending hands toward feet as much or as little as feels good on legs and lower back. Allow your head to relax down toward your legs. (If hamstrings are tight, soften knees.) Breath here for as long as it feels good.

When you are ready to come out, one vertebra at a time, roll up and then onto back, keeping soft knees. Bend knees and place feet on the floor with arms on either side. Soften knees and press arms into the ground to reach feet up toward the ceiling. Breath here for as long as it is comfortable.

When you feel comfortable, allow feet to fall back behind you an amount that feels good on your neck.

Reach feet to the ground for plough pose. Clasp hands together on the ground and wiggle shoulders underneath you one at a time. Press firmly into arms, reach through heels, and breath here for at least three deep breaths.

To come down, slowly soften knees toward forehead, come back to plough, and slowly lower back to mat one vertebra at a time.

ANXIETY

Anxiety is caused by not knowing what is going on, usually lack of knowledge about something. Knowing the issue is half the battle, because you at least have some way of knowing how to tackle it. When you are anxious, you are unable to think clearly and your mind is fuddled with mixed messages. You seek advice from others who are even less clued up about situations than you and find yourself with even more voices in your head. Yoga clears the mind, calms the spirit, and makes you do the right action both within the posture and out of it. There will be times when you will wish you could do yoga all day because it is then you are at your most calm because you are in a meditative state.

These postures help with that meditative state. It is not about doing them 'right', it is about aligning yourself in the posture and breathing deeply and slowly and regularly from your abdominals, not your chest. Don't get 'anxious' about doing the postures right or wrong.

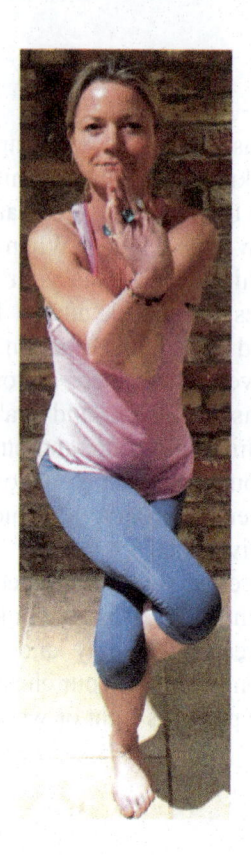

EAGLE POSE OR GARUDASANA

This wonderful balancing posture quietens the mind and brings attention to the body. Try holding the pose for sixty seconds on each side. This is a warming and balancing yoga posture which strengthens your thighs, ankles and calves, stretches your shoulders, arms and upper back and develops focus and concentration as it improves your balance and coordination.

STEP BY STEP

Stand in Tadasana. Bend your knees slightly, lift your left foot up and, balancing on your right foot, cross your left thigh over the right. Point your left toes toward the floor, press the foot back, and then hook the top of the foot behind the lower right calf. Balance on the right foot.

Stretch your arms straight forward, parallel to the floor, and spread your scapulas wide across the back of your torso.

Cross the arms in front of your torso so that the right arm is above the left, then bend your elbows. Snug the right elbow into the crook of the left, and raise your forearms perpendicular to the floor. The backs of your hands should be facing each other.

Press the right hand to the right and the left hand to the left, so that the palms are now facing each other. The thumb of the right hand should pass in front of the little finger of the left. Now press the palms together (as much as is possible for you), lift your elbows up, and stretch the fingers toward the ceiling.

Stay for 15 to 30 seconds, then unwind the legs and arms and stand in Tadasana again. Repeat for the same length of time with the arms and legs reversed.

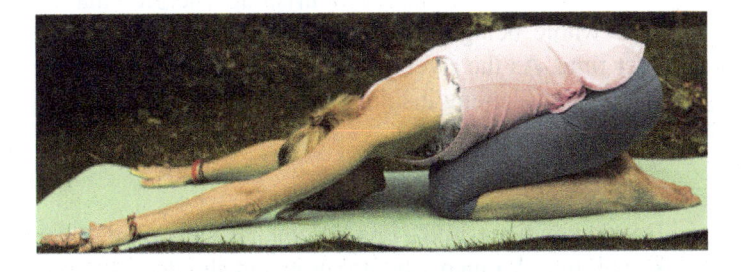

CHILD POSE OR BALASANA

One of the main resting poses of yoga practice, child's pose involves sitting on the knees and bending forward with arms forward or by your side. It is comforting and self-soothing. It slows the mind and helps us focus on the breath. This asana gently stretches your lower back, hips, thighs, knees, and ankles, relaxes your spine, shoulders and neck increases blood circulation to your head which reduces headaches, massages your internal organs, calms the mind (central nervous system) thus helping relieve stress and tension.

With the innocence and unselfconsciousness of a small child, rest your upper body along your upper thighs as your hips melt down toward your heels.

Allow your forehead to find its support on the Earth as you feel nurtured and protected at the same time. In this safe space, with your eyes closed and your gaze internally focused, become aware of the grief pangs which are residing in your heart.

Who has passed from your life? Which relationship have you lost? What sadness remains?

As you breath deeply into your child body, let your heart open the door into your emotional field and observe what lies within you. The child is faithful in each moment to whatever emotion is awake and alive. Be the child, feeling fully and not holding anything back.

Cry if the tears come streaming down. Let memories of that which has passed flood your being.

Mother yourself in the nourishing energies that relax your whole being and soften the grief that has hardened over time. As the river of grief is liberated, feel a sense of freedom awakening inside you.

STEP BY STEP

Do not practice Child's Pose if you have a current or recent knee injury. Women who are pregnant should only practice a wide-legged variation of the pose — do not press the belly on top of the thighs.

Always work within your own range of limits and abilities. If you have any medical concerns, talk with your doctor before practicing yoga.

Begin on your hands and knees. Centre your breath, and begin to let your thoughts slow down. Turn your awareness inward. Spread your knees wide apart while keeping your big toes touching. Rest your buttocks on your heels. Those with very tight hips can keep their knees and thighs together.

Sit up straight and lengthen your spine up through the crown of your head.

On an exhalation, bow forward, draping your torso between your thighs. Your heart and chest should rest between or on top of your thighs. Allow your forehead to come to the floor. Keep your arms long and extended, palms facing down.

Press back slightly with your hands to keep your buttocks in contact with your heels.

Lengthen from your hips to your armpits, and then extend even further through your fingertips. For deeper relaxation, bring your arms back to rest alongside your thighs with your palms facing up. Completely relax your elbows.

Let your upper back broaden. Soften and relax your lower back. Allow all tension in your shoulders, arms, and neck to drain away. Keep your gaze drawn inward with your eyes closed. Hold for up to a minute or longer, breathing softly.

To release the pose, gently use your hands to walk your torso upright to sit back on your heels.

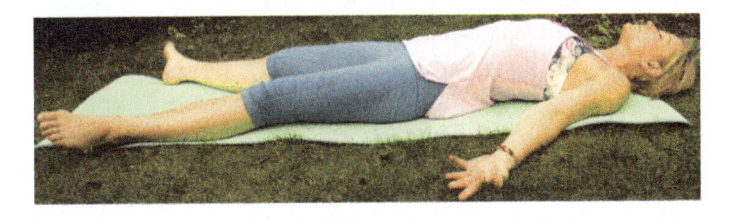

CORPSE POSE OR SAVASANA

Savasana is appropriate for all yoga students. If you are uncomfortable lying on your back, practice a supported version of the pose. Women who are pregnant should keep their head and chest raised in the pose by resting on a bolster or cushion. Always work within your own range of limits and abilities. If you have any medical concerns, talk with your doctor before practicing yoga.

STEP BY STEP

Lie on your back with your legs straight and arms at your sides. Rest your hands about six inches away from your body with your palms up. Let your feet drop open. Close your eyes. You may want to cover your body with a blanket.

Let your breath occur naturally. Allow your body to feel heavy on the ground. Working from the soles of your feet up to the crown of your head, consciously release every body part, organ, and cell.

Relax your face. Let your eyes drop deep into their sockets. Invite peace and silence into your mind, body, and soul. Stay in Savasana for five minutes for every 30 minutes of your practice.

To exit the pose, first begin to deepen your breath. Bring gentle movement and awareness back to your body, wiggling your fingers and toes. Roll to your right side and rest there for a moment. With an inhalation, gently press yourself into a comfortable seated position. Let your head be the last thing to come into place. Carry the peace and stillness of Savasana with you throughout the rest of your day.

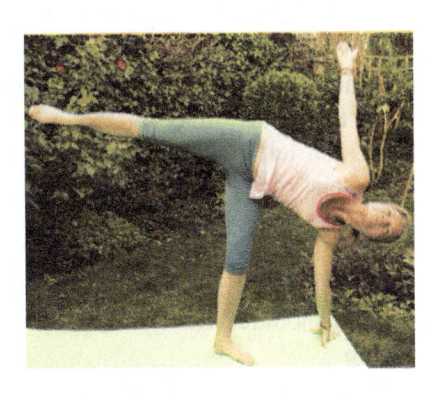

HALF MOON POSE OR ARDHA CHANDRASANA

This asana quiets the mind, yet brings awareness. Half Moon is a balancing posture with one leg raised 90 degrees and one hand on the floor or on a block. Balancing poses take our attention from our mind and into our body, expands your chest and shoulders, increases mobility of your hip joints, increases neck mobility, lengthens your spinal muscles, strengthens and tones the muscles of your thighs and calves, stretches your hamstrings and groin muscles and increases proprioception (the sense of position in space) of the feet and ankles.

STEP BY STEP

Do not practice Half Moon Pose if you have low blood pressure or are currently experiencing headaches, insomnia, or diarrhoea. Those with neck injuries should not turn their heads to face the top hand, but should continue looking straight ahead. Always work within your own range of limits and abilities. If you have any medical concerns, talk with your doctor before practicing yoga.

Begin by standing at the top of your mat. Turn to the left and step your feet wide apart. Extend your arms out to the sides at shoulder-height. Your feet should be as far apart as your wrists. Rotate your right (front) foot 90 degrees, so your front foot's toes point to the top of the mat. Turn your left foot's toes slightly in. Align your front heel with the arch of your back foot. Reach through your right hand in the same direction that your right foot is pointed. Shift your left hip back, and then fold sideways at the hip. Rest your right hand on your outer right shin or ankle. If you are more flexible, place your fingertips on the floor. You can also place your hand on a block.

Align your shoulders so your left shoulder is directly above your right shoulder. Gently turn your head to gaze at your left thumb.

Bring your left hand to rest on your left hip. Turn your head to look at the floor. Then bend your right knee and step your left foot 6-12 inches closer to your right foot. Place your right hand's fingertips on the floor in front of your right foot.

Press firmly into your right hand and foot. Straighten your right leg while simultaneously lifting your left leg. Work toward bringing your left leg parallel to the floor, or even higher than your hips.

Reach actively through your left heel. Do not lock your right leg's knee. Keep your right foot's toes and kneecap facing in the direction of your head.

Stack your top hip directly over your bottom hip, and open your torso to the left. Then extend your left arm and point your fingertips directly toward the sky. If you can balance comfortably there, turn your head and gaze at your left thumb.

Draw your shoulder blades firmly into your back. Lengthen your tailbone toward your left heel.

Hold for up to one minute. To release, lower your left leg as you exhale. Return to Extended Triangle Pose. Inhale and press firmly through your left heel as you lift your torso. Lower your arms. Turn to the left, reversing the position of your feet, and repeat for the same length of time on the opposite side.

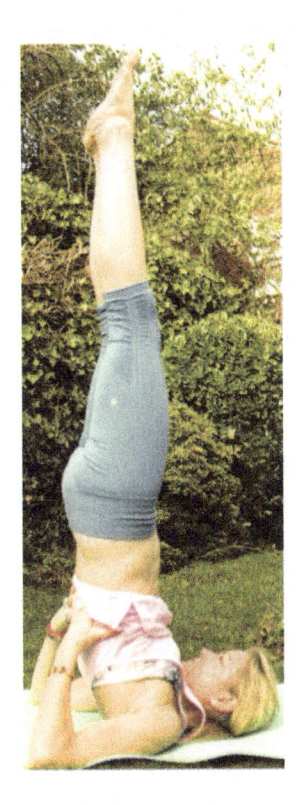

SUPPORTED SHOULDER STAND OR SALAMBA SARVANGASANA

Inversions help you get out of the 'monkey mind' by putting you in a different position to normal life They literally turn things upside down, and stress and anxiety are a perception of danger and unease, and when you can get out of your mind – that helps. This posture tones your legs, buttocks, back and core muscles, stretches your shoulders and improves flexibility of your upper spine.

It also calms the brain and nervous system, therefore helping to relieve stress, improves digestion and massages and stimulates the thyroid and prostate glands and flushes mucous from your lungs.

Inversions help you get out of the 'monkey mind' by putting you in a different position to normal life They literally turn things up side down, and stress and anxiety are a perception of danger and unease, and when you can get out of your mind - that helps.

STEP BY STEP

Begin in a seated position with legs extended long and together and arms relaxed on either side. Take a big inhale. On the exhalation, fall forward, pulling navel to spine and extending hands toward feet as much or as little as feels good on the legs and lower back. Allow head to relax down toward legs. (If hamstrings are tight, soften knees.) Breath here for as long as it feels good.

When you are ready to come out, one vertebra at a time, roll up and then onto back, keeping soft knees. Bend knees and place feet on the floor with arms on either side. Soften knees and press arms into the ground to reach feet up toward the ceiling. Breath here for as long as is comfortable.

When you feel comfortable, allow feet to fall back behind you an amount that feels good on your neck.

Reach feet to the ground for plough pose. Clasp hands together on the ground and wiggle shoulders underneath you one at a time. Press firmly into arms, reach through heels, and breath here for at least three deep breaths.

From plough or modified plough, place hands on lower back for support and try to keep elbows about shoulder-width apart. Soften legs and allow knees to rest on forehead in an egg shape. Breath here for as long as it is comfortable.

When you feel steady, reach feet toward ceiling one at a time, lengthening legs when you feel comfortable. Breath here for at least three deep breaths. To come down, slowly soften knees toward forehead, come back to plough, and slowly lower back to mat one vertebra at a time.

Fish pose is a great counterpart to shoulder stand and can be an effective way to relieve neck and back pain, improve circulation, and open your chest muscles.

Place hands and palms underneath butt and hips. Keep elbows as close together as possible and fingertips facing forward with forearms parallel to each other on the ground. Bend elbows and lean onto forearms, pressing them into the floor. Lift chest up toward the ceiling so that back is arched. Bring elbows toward each other until they're about shoulder-width apart. Allow head to relax down toward the ground until it touches the mat. Breath here for at least three deep breaths. When ready, come out of this slowly and lie on your back for a few breaths to enjoy how great you feel.

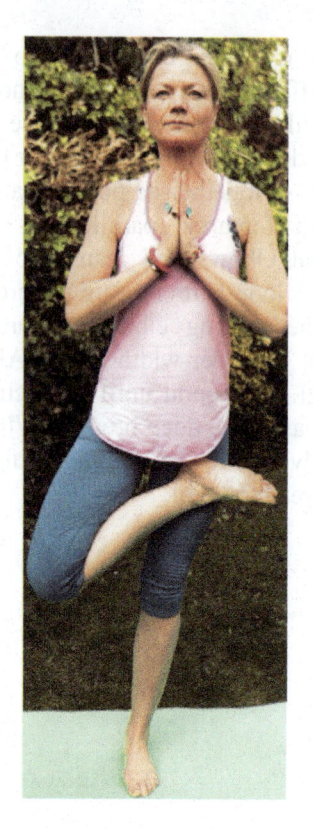

TREE POSE OR VRKSASANA

This asana forces you to be honest about where you are currently not being honest. If you are in a tree pose and your mind is wandering – you will fall over. Try this before you try Eagle and Half Moon pose. This posture stretches your inner thighs, groin and shoulders strengthens your thighs, calves, core and foot muscles, strengthens your posture, calms and relaxes your mind and central nervous system, develops balance and increases your mind/body awareness.

STEP BY STEP

Improves focus and sense of balance. Supports a feeling of connection with the Earth and current environment.

Starting in mountain pose begin to shift weight into left foot, bending right knee to bring your right foot and ankle to your calf or inner thigh of left leg.

Focus eyes on the Earth three to five feet in front of you. If you have a hard time balancing, rest one or both hands against a wall. Encourage both hips to be in a neutral position, parallel to the floor.

Bring palms to touch at your heart's centre, interlacing middle, ring and pinkie fingers leaving index fingers and thumbs extended. Press left foot firmly into the ground.

Inhale and extend arms overhead, lengthening up. Hold for eight to ten diaphragmatic breaths, then on an exhale return to mountain pose and repeat on opposite side.

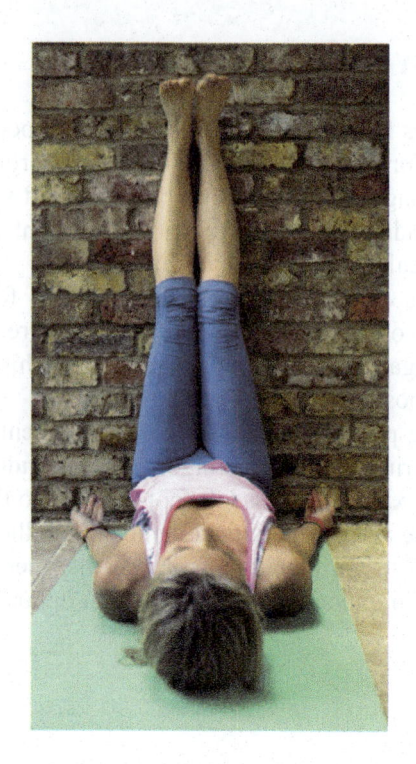

LEGS UP THE WALL POSE OR VIPARITA KARANI

This asana helps you escape the 'thinking mind'. You don't need to be so flexible or so strong, and yet it's very relaxing and very calming of the nervous system. This posture is restorative, relaxing and a gentle inversion that has many benefits. It eases anxiety and stress, is therapeutic for arthritis, headaches, high blood pressure, low blood pressure and insomnia, eases symptoms of premenstrual syndrome, menstrual cramps and menopause, relieves tired or cramped feet and legs, gently stretches the hamstrings, legs and lower back, relieves lower back pain and calms the mind.

STEP BY STEP

The pose described here is a passive, supported variation of the Shoulder Stand–like Viparita Karani. For your support you'll need one or two thickly folded blankets or a firm round bolster. You'll also need to rest your legs vertically (or nearly so) on a wall or other upright support.

Before performing the pose, determine two things about your support: its height and its distance from the wall. If you're stiff, the support should be lower and placed further from the wall; if you're more flexible, use a higher support that is closer to the wall. Your distance from the wall also depends on your height: if you're shorter move closer to the wall, if taller move further from the wall. Experiment with the position of your support until you find the placement that works for you.

Start with your support about five to six inches away from the wall. Sit sideways on the right end of the support, with your right side against the wall (left-handers can substitute "left" for "right" in these instructions).

Exhale and, with one smooth movement, swing your legs up onto the wall and your shoulders and head lightly down onto the floor. The first few times you do this, you may ignominiously slide off the support and plop down with your buttocks on the floor.

Don't get discouraged. Try lowering the support and/or moving it slightly further off the wall until you gain some facility with this movement, then move back closer to the wall. Your sitting bones don't need to be right against the wall, but they should be "dripping" down into the space between the support and the wall.

Check that the front of your torso gently arches from the pubis to the top of the shoulders. If the front of your torso seems flat, then you've probably slipped a bit off the support. Bend your knees, press your feet into the wall and lift your pelvis off the support a few inches, tuck the support a little higher up under your pelvis, then lower your pelvis onto the support again.

Lift and release the base of your skull away from the back of your neck and soften your throat. Don't push your chin against your sternum; instead let your sternum lift toward the chin. Take a small roll (made from a towel for example) under your neck if the cervical spine feels flat.

Open your shoulder blades away from the spine and release your hands and arms out to your sides, palms up. Keep your legs relatively firm, just enough to hold them vertically in place.

Release the heads of the thigh bones and the weight of your belly deeply into your torso, toward the back of the pelvis.

Soften your eyes and turn them down to look into your heart. Stay in this pose anywhere from five to fifteen minutes. Be sure not to twist off the support when coming out. Instead, slide off the support onto the floor before turning to the side.

You can also bend your knees and push your feet against the wall to lift your pelvis off the support. Then slide the support to one side, lower your pelvis to the floor, and turn to the side.

Stay on your side for a few breaths, and come up to sitting with an exhalation.

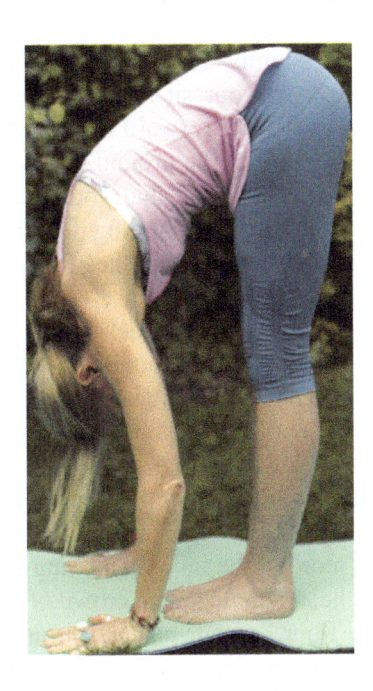

STANDING FORWARD BEND OR UTTANASANA

Forward bends are excellent for calming our nervous system. The posture provides a release of the upper body and soothes the mind through gentle inversion, either when practiced on its own or between postures. This posture stretches your hips, hamstrings and calves, strengthens your thighs and knees, massages your internal organs and helps improve digestion and cleanses mucus from the lungs, relaxes your central nervous system and helps calm your mind, helps relieve stress, headaches, fatigue and insomnia; helps relieve symptoms of menopause and is therapeutic for osteoporosis.

As you stand in Mountain Pose (Tadasana), place your hands on your hips and inhale. As you exhale, soften your knees and fold slowly forward from your hips. Counterbalance your body weight by moving your tailbone

and hips back slightly as the body leans forward. Keep your knees soft so your sit bones point up to the ceiling and your hip points roll forward into the upper thighs.

Rest your hands on the ground beside your feet or hold onto your elbows. Ensure that your feet are still parallel (second and midde toes pointing forward). Hollow out your belly and encourage the chest bone to float down to the top of your feet and increase the space between your pubis and your chest bone. Feel that the fold comes from your hip joint and not from rounding of your lower back.

If the hamstrings feel ease in this stretch, slowly extend your knees more while pushing your sit bones up to the ceiling.

Root into the heels as you lightly turn the top of the thighs inwards. This inwards rotation of your thighs aligns and isolates more of the inner hamstring lines.

Let your head dangle so the crown of your head reaches down to the floor so your gaze is through the legs. Hold for several slow breaths.

To exit, contract your abdominal and core muscles.

As you inhale, place your hands on your hips, soften your knees, and reach your chest far forward. Rise up from your hips keeping your back long. Keep the length between the pubis and chest bone. Continue to lengthen your torso as you come up to standing.

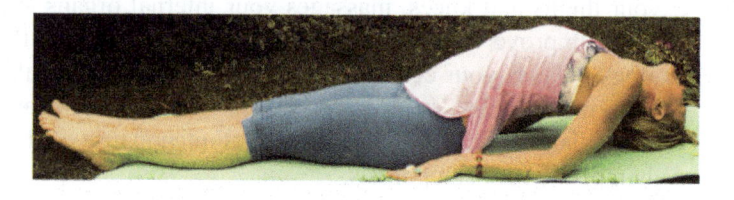

FISH POSE OR MATSYASANA

This particular posture is usually practiced following the Shoulder Stand as a counter-balance. After turning your world upside down, it's now time to focus on expanding and opening the heart and lung area. Fear often settles in this area, creating a kind of static that keeps us from being able to clearly hear our loving inner voice.

As your body weight rests on your legs, buttocks, forearms and the crown of the head, lift the rib cage and upper chest area as high as it will go upward. Create an opening directly from your heart...

Place a thickly folded blanket beneath the head for support if you are experiencing discomfort.

This pose opens your pectorals, the muscles of your chest, the intercostal muscles between your ribs, and the upper portion of psoas muscles in your hips, improves the quality of your breath by opening the accessory muscles of breathing, opens muscles in your abdomen and in the front of your neck, relieves thoracic and mid back spinal tension, strengthens musculature in your back and neck, and is traditionally thought to stimulate organs in the abdomen and throat.

STEP BY STEP

Lie on your back on the floor with your knees bent, feet on the floor. Inhale, lift your pelvis slightly off the floor, and slide your hands, palms down, below your buttocks. Then rest your buttocks on the backs of your hands (and don't lift them off your hands as you perform this pose). Be sure to tuck your forearms and elbows up close to the sides of your torso. Inhale and press your forearms and elbows firmly against the floor. Next press your scapulas into your back and, with an inhale, lift your upper torso and head away from the floor. Then release your head back onto the floor. Depending on how high you arch your back and lift your chest, either the back of your head or its crown will rest on the floor. There should be a minimal amount of weight on your head to avoid crunching your neck.

You can keep your knees bent or straighten your legs out onto the floor. If you do the latter, keep your thighs active, and press out through the heels. Stay for 15 to 30 seconds, breathing smoothly. With an exhalation, lower your torso and head to the floor. Draw your thighs up into your belly and squeeze.

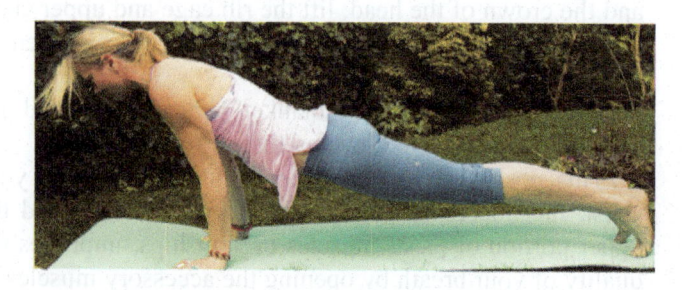

PLANK POSE OR PHALAKASANA

This posture strengthens and tones the entire body, with particular focus on the arms, wrists, shoulders and abdomen. It builds endurance and spinal support by strengthening the core muscles, aiding a better posture.

STEP BY STEP

Start in Downward Dog posture. Then inhale and draw your torso forward until the arms are perpendicular to the floor and the shoulders directly over the wrists, torso parallel to the floor.

Press your outer arms inward and firm the bases of your index fingers into the floor. Firm your shoulder blades against your back, then spread them away from the spine. Also spread your collarbones away from the sternum.

Press your front thighs up toward the ceiling, but resist your tailbone toward the floor as you lengthen it toward the heels. Lift the base of the skull away from the back of the neck and look straight down at the floor, keeping the throat and eyes soft.

Plank Pose is one of the positions in the traditional Sun Salutation sequence. You can also perform this pose by itself and stay anywhere from 30 seconds to one minute.

HEARTBREAK

You can't get them out of your mind. And your heart hurts. There's a tightness in your ribcage, and you don't want to eat. You can't do anything and the pain is so intense it wakes you up in the middle of the night. And no matter what logic you use, how many self help books you read, you are in pain and you want it to go away. Knowing men love women differently, and that happiness never comes from love of another – and that only the love between that of a mother and child is unconditional – or should be – will hopefully help women understand why they should never sleep with someone until the man is 'committed' in some way (financially, emotionally, mentally), although they will never be truly committed. But don't blame them. It's a bit like criticising an apple for not being a pear.

Yoga releases dormant, emotional energy, which can help you confront unresolved issues. Heartbreak and depression linger in the chest, while anger and frustration can cause spinal tension. Incorporating these yoga poses into your daily heartbreak regime will be a strong step forward.

Everyone has advice on heartbreak. Yoga philosophies also offer advice, which I've edited here in bullet points.

Don't judge yourself to be not good enough for this person. You are amazing, always remember that, even if the other person has forgotten it.

Don't doubt yourself.

Are you mourning their loss or is the feeling of being rejected? They are not the same.

They did not make you happy – you make you happy.

Be grateful and contented with the other people in your life. They recognise you for who you are. Recognise those who love you conditionally and those who do not.

This one is tough. Trust that the universe knows what it is doing. That everything is for the best. You are on the path you are meant to be. It is extremely painful at the moment but it will pass. A lot of people take up yoga during divorce, bereavement, midlife crisis – in their 40s and 50s because they realise what they want is not what they have spent the past forty or so years searching for. It is not fame or fortune. It is PEACE and LOVE. That is essentially what all human beings want.

You can apply logic as much as you like, talk as much as you like, cry as much as you like.

Last thing. **There is a line in the film 'Dangerous Liaisons' which is spot on where heartbreak is concerned.**

"Men do not love the way women do. They are not capable of loving one person exclusively. That has always been the case. Men are made happy by the love they feel. Women are made happy by the love they give. So any woman who wishes to be made happy by love is going to be disappointed by it."

In other words, don't base your happiness on a relationship with anyone or anything external to you. Base it on the relationship you have with yourself.

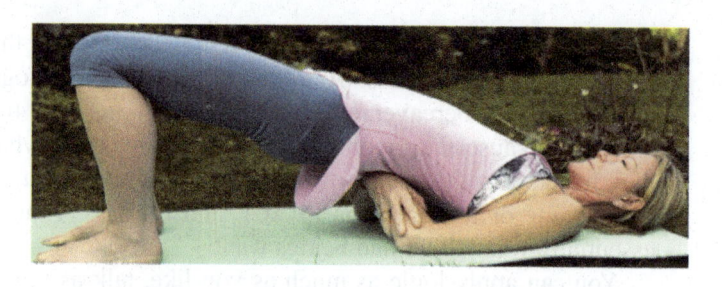

BRIDGE POSE OR SETU BANDHASANA

This posture stretches your chest, neck and spine and hips, strengthens your back, buttocks, and hamstring muscles, calms your brain and central nervous system, which helps alleviate stress and midl depression, massages abdominal organs and improves digestion, stimulates the lungs and thyroid glands and helps relieve the symptoms of menopause, reduces anxiety, backache, headache and insomnia. Heart openers might be the last thing anyone wants to do after a heartbreak, however it should be a priority to not keep negative emotion in the chest. The Bridge pose is a gentle way to release emotions. The chest opening isn't as striking as camel pose, but it still makes a difference.

STEP BY STEP

Do not perform this pose if you have a neck or shoulder injury. Always work within your own range of limits and abilities. If you have any medical concerns, talk with your doctor before practicing yoga.

Lie on your back with your knees bent and feet on the floor. Extend your arms along the floor, palms flat.

Press your feet and arms firmly into the floor. Exhale as you lift your hips toward the ceiling. Draw your tailbone toward your pubic bone, holding your buttocks off the floor. Do not squeeze your glutes or flex your buttocks.

Roll your shoulders back and underneath your body. Clasp your hands and extend your arms along the floor beneath your pelvis. Straighten your arms as much as possible, pressing your forearms into the mat. Reach your knuckles toward your heels.

Keep your thighs and feet parallel — do not roll to the outer edges of your feet or let your knees drop together.

Press your weight evenly across all four corners of both feet. Lengthen your tailbone toward the backs of your knees. Hold for up to one minute.

To release, unclasp your hands and place them palms-down alongside your body. Exhale as you slowly roll your spine along the floor, vertebra by vertebra. Allow your knees to drop together.

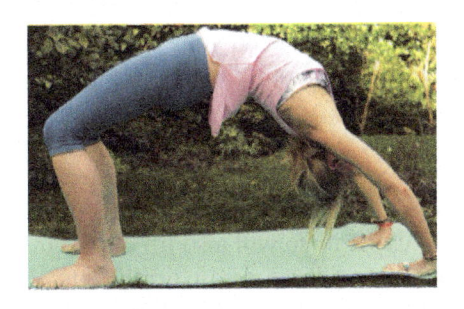

FULL WHEEL POSE OR URDHVA DHANURASANA

This asana expands your chest and shoulders, stretches your hip flexors and core muscles, stretches your wrist flexor muscles and strengthens the muscles that control your shoulder blades.

STEP BY STEP

Do not practice this pose if you are currently experiencing high or low blood pressure, headaches, diarrhoea, or heart problems. Also avoid this pose if you have a back injury or carpal tunnel syndrome.

Upward Bow requires a great deal of strength and flexibility to be performed correctly. It is very easy to injure yourself if you attempt to move into it too soon, if you do not yet have the strength or flexibility to do the pose in correct alignment.

Do not practice this pose if you are currently experiencing high or low blood pressure, migraines, or insomnia. Also avoid this pose if you are pregnant, or if you have a lower back or neck injury.

Always work within your own range of limits and abilities. If you have any medical concerns, talk with your doctor before practicing yoga. Begin by lying flat on your stomach with your chin on the mat and your hands resting at your sides.

On an exhalation, bend your knees. Bring your heels as close as you can to your buttocks, keeping your knees hip-distance apart.

Reach back with both hands and hold onto your outer ankles. On an inhalation, lift your heels up toward the ceiling, drawing your thighs up and off the mat. Your head, chest, and upper torso will also lift off the mat.

Draw your tailbone down firmly into the floor, while you simultaneously lift your heels and thighs even higher.

Lift your chest and press your shoulder blades firmly into your upper back. Draw your shoulders away from your ears. Gaze forward and breath softly. Your breath will become shallow, but do not hold your breath.

Hold for up to 30 seconds. To release, exhale and gently lower your thighs to the mat. Slowly release your legs and feet to the floor. Place your right ear on the mat and relax your arms at your sides for a few breaths. Repeat the pose for the same amount of time, then rest with your left ear on the mat.

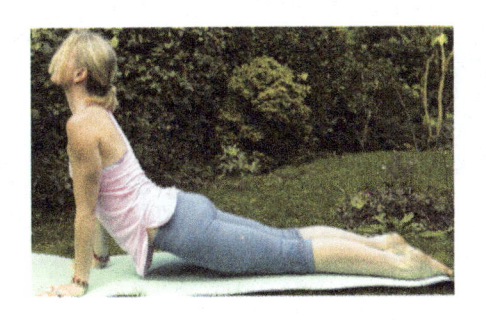

COBRA POSE OR BHUJANGASANA

This posture strengthens your back muscles and arms, increases the flexibility of your spine, stretches your chest, shoulders, lungs, and abdomen, stretches and massages your internal organs and firms your buttocks.

STEP BY STEP

Lie prone on the floor. Stretch your legs back, tops of the feet on the floor. Spread your hands on the floor under your shoulders. Hug the elbows back into your body.

Press the tops of the feet and thighs and the pubis firmly into the floor.

On an inhalation, begin to straighten the arms to lift the chest off the floor, going only to the height at which you can maintain a connection through your pubis to your legs. Press the tailbone toward the pubis and lift the pubis toward the navel. Narrow the hip points. Firm but don't harden the buttocks.

Firm the shoulder blades against the back, puffing the side ribs forward. Lift through the top of the sternum but avoid pushing the front ribs forward, which only hardens the lower back. Distribute the backbend evenly throughout the entire spine.

Hold the pose anywhere from 15 to 30 seconds, breathing easily. Release back to the floor with an exhalation.

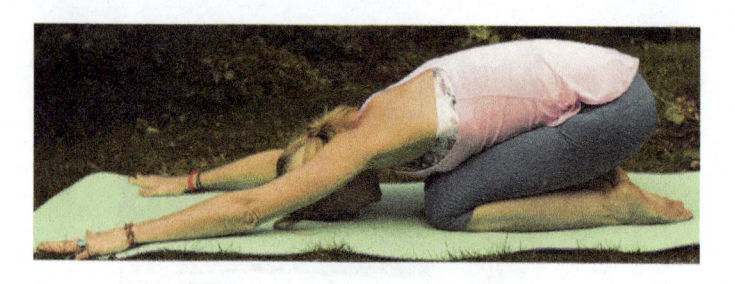

CHILD POSE OR BALASANA

One of the main resting poses of yoga practice, child's pose involves sitting on the knees and bending forward with arms forward or by your side. It is comforting and self-soothing. It slows the mind and helps us focus on the breath. The asana gently stretches your lower back, hips, thighs, knees, and ankles, relaxes your spine, shoulders and neck increases blood circulation to your head which reduces headaches, massages your internal organs and calms the mind (central nervous system), thus helping relieve stress and tension.

With the innocence and unselfconsciousness of a small child, rest your upper body along your upper thighs as your hips melt down toward your heels. Allow your forehead to find its support on the Earth as you feel nurtured and protected at the same time. In this safe space, with your eyes closed and your gaze internally focused, become aware of the grief pangs which are residing in your heart.

Who has passed from your life? Which relationship have you lost? What sadness remains?

As you breath deeply into your child body, let your heart open the door into your emotional field and observe what lies within you. The child is faithful in each moment to whatever emotion is awake and alive. Be the child, feeling fully and not holding anything back. Cry if the tears come streaming down. Let memories of that which has passed flood your being. Mother yourself in the nourishing energies that relax your whole being and soften the grief that has hardened over time. As the river of grief is liberated, feel a sense of freedom awakening inside you.

STEP BY STEP

Do not practice Child's Pose if you have a current or recent knee injury. Women who are pregnant should only practice a wide-legged variation of the pose — do not press the belly on top of the thighs.

Always work within your own range of limits and abilities. If you have any medical concerns, talk with your doctor before practicing yoga.

Begin on your hands and knees. Centre your breath, and begin to let your thoughts slow down. Turn your awareness inward. Spread your knees wide apart while keeping your big toes touching. Rest your buttocks on your heels. Those with very tight hips can keep their knees and thighs together.

Sit up straight and lengthen your spine up through the crown of your head. On an exhalation, bow forward, draping your torso between your thighs. Your heart and chest should rest between or on top of your thighs.

Allow your forehead to come to the floor. Keep your arms long and extended, palms facing down. Press back slightly with your hands to keep your buttocks in contact with your heels. Lengthen from your hips to your armpits, and then extend even further through your fingertips. For deeper relaxation, bring your arms back to rest alongside your thighs with your palms facing up. Completely relax your elbows. Let your upper back broaden. Soften and relax your lower back. Allow all tension in your shoulders, arms, and neck to drain away.

Keep your gaze drawn inward with your eyes closed. Hold for up to a minute or longer, breathing softly. To release the pose, gently use your hands to walk your torso upright to sit back on your heels.

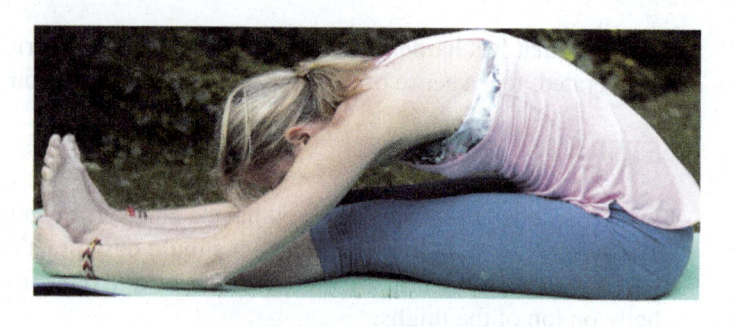

SEATED FORWARD BEND OR PASCHIMOTTANASANA

This asana stretches the hamstring, spine and lower back, calms the mind and relieves stress and anxiety, improves digestion, relieves symptoms of PMS and menopause, reduces fatigue and stimulates the liver, kidneys, ovaries, and uterus. Forward and backbends are great for removing anger, betrayal and all other negative emotions that cause spinal tension. This pose also helps increase awareness by releasing energies that cloud clear thought.

STEP BY STEP

Begin in a seated position with legs extended long and together and arms relaxed on either side. Take a big inhalation. On the exhalation, fall forward, pulling navel to spine and extending hands toward feet as much or as little as feels good on legs and lower back. Allow head to relax down toward legs. (If hamstrings are tight, soften knees.) Breath here for as long as it feels good.

When you are ready to come out, one vertebra at a time, roll up and then onto back, keeping soft knees. Bend knees and place feet on the floor with arms on either side. Soften knees and press arms into the ground to reach feet up toward the ceiling. Breath here for as long as is comfortable.

When you feel comfortable, allow feet to fall back behind you an amount that feels good on your neck.

Reach feet to the ground for plough pose. Clasp hands together on the ground and wiggle shoulders underneath you one at a time. Press firmly into arms, reach through heels, and breath here for at least three deep breaths.

From plough or modified plough, place hands on lower back for support and try to keep elbows about shoulder-width apart. Soften legs and allow knees to rest on forehead. Breath here for as long as it is comfortable.

When you feel steady, reach feet toward the ceiling one at a time, lengthening legs when you feel comfortable. Breath here for at least three deep breaths. To come down, slowly soften knees toward forehead, come back to plough, and slowly lower back to mat one vertebra at a time.

Fish pose is a great counterpart to shoulder stand and can be an effective way to relieve neck and back pain, improve circulation, and open your chest muscles.

Place hands and palms underneath butt and hips. Keep elbows as close together as possible and fingertips facing forward with forearms parallel to each other on the ground. Bend elbows and lean onto forearms, pressing them into the floor. Lift chest up toward the ceiling so that back is arched. Bring elbows toward each other until they're about shoulder-width apart. Allow head to relax down toward the ground until it touches the mat. Breath here for at least three deep breaths. When ready, come out of this slowly and lie on your back for a few breaths to enjoy how great you feel.

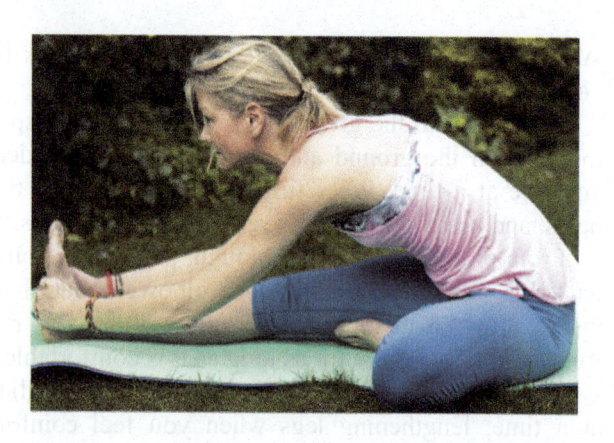

KNEE TO HEAD POSE OR JANU SIRSASANA

This posture stretches your spine, back muscles, hamstrings and groin, massages and stimulates your internal organs like the liver and kidneys, improves digestion and helps heal gastric ailments and calms the mind and central nervous system.

STEP BY STEP

Avoid practicing this pose if you are currently suffering from asthma or diarrhoea. Students with back or knee injuries should only practice this pose with the guidance of an experienced and knowledgeable teacher.

Always work within your own range of limits and abilities. If you have any medical concerns, talk with your doctor before practicing yoga.

Sit on the edge of a firm blanket, with your legs extended in front of you in Staff Pose (Dandasana). Bring the sole of your left foot to the inside of your right thigh. Align the centre of your torso with your right leg (a mild twist).

Keeping your spine long, exhale as you hinge forward from the hips to fold over your right leg. Imagine your torso coming to rest on your right thigh, rather than reaching your nose toward your knee (so bend at your waist).

Draw your right thigh down and flex your foot. Hold onto your right leg's shin, ankle, or foot. You can also wrap a yoga strap or towel around the sole of your right foot and hold it firmly with both hands. Keep the front of your torso long; do not round your back. Let your belly touch your thigh first, and then your chest. Your head and nose should touch your leg last.

With each inhalation, lengthen the front torso.

With each exhalation, fold deeper. Hold for 30 seconds. To release the pose, draw your tailbone toward the floor as you inhale and lift your torso. Extend your left leg.

Repeat the pose on the opposite side.

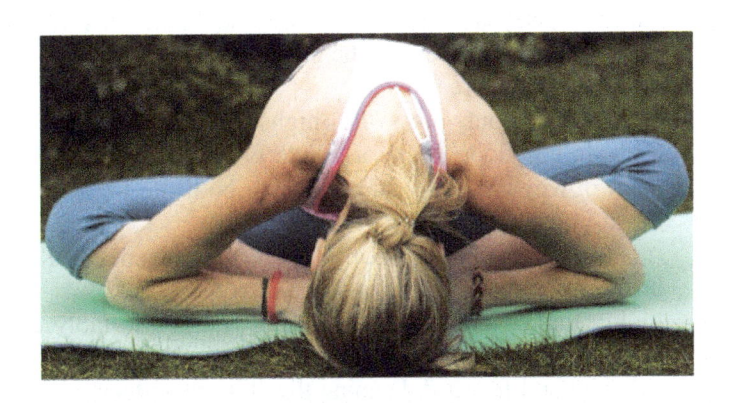

BOUND ANGLE POSE/BUTTERFLY POSE OR BADDHA KONASANA

This asana stretches and expands your inner thigh, groin and knee muscles, stretches your lower back and upper gluteal muscles when you are in the forward bend variation, massages your abdominal organs and improves digestive circulation.

STEP BY STEP

The posture is named Baddha Konasana because of the way it is carried out – both the feet tucked close to the groin, clasped tightly with the hands as though tied or bound together in a particular angle. It is also popularly known as the Butterfly Pose because of the movement of the legs during the posture, giving the appearance of a butterfly flapping its wings.

The posture is also sometimes known as the Cobbler Pose as it resembles the sitting position of a cobbler at work.

How to do Butterfly Pose (Baddha Konasana):

Sit with your spine erect and legs spread straight out. Now bend your knees and bring your feet towards the pelvis. The soles of your feet should touch each other. Grab your feet tightly with your hands. You may place the hands underneath the feet for support. Make an effort to bring the heels as close to the genitals as possible.

Take a deep breath in.

Breathing out, press the thighs and knees downward towards the floor. Make a gentle effort to keep pressing them downward. Now start flapping both the legs up and down like the wings of a butterfly.

Start slow and gradually increase the speed. Keep breathing normally throughout.

Fly higher and higher, as fast as you comfortably can. Slow down and then stop. Take a deep breath in and as you exhale, bend forward, keeping the chin up and spine erect. Press your elbows on the thighs or on the knees, pushing the knees and thighs closer to the floor.

Feel the stretch in the inner thighs and take long, deep breaths, relaxing the muscles more and more. Take a deep breath in and bring the torso up. As you exhale, gently release the posture.

Straighten the legs out in front of you and relax.

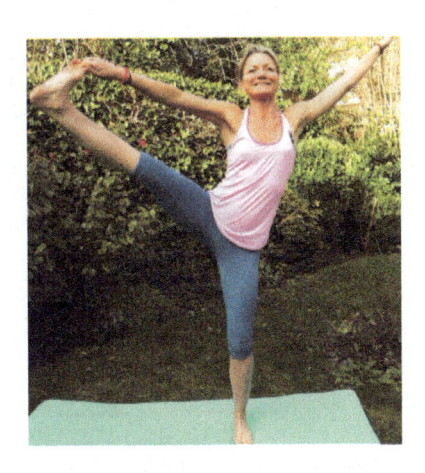

EXTENDED HAND TO TOE POSE OR UTTHITA HASTA PADANGUSTHASANA

This posture stretches hamstrings and hips, strengthens back and arm muscles, improves sense of balance, calms the mind and improves focus.

STEP BY STEP

From Tadasana, bring your left knee toward your belly. Reach your left arm inside the thigh, cross it over the front ankle, and hold the outside of your left foot. If your hamstrings are tight, hold a strap looped around the left sole.

Firm the front thigh muscles of the standing leg, and press the outer thigh inward.

Inhale and extend the left leg forward. Straighten the knee as much as possible. If you're steady, swing the leg out to the side. Breath steadily; breathing takes concentration, but it helps you balance.

Hold for 30 seconds, then swing the leg back to centre with an inhale, and lower the foot to the floor with an exhale. Repeat on the other side for the same length of time.

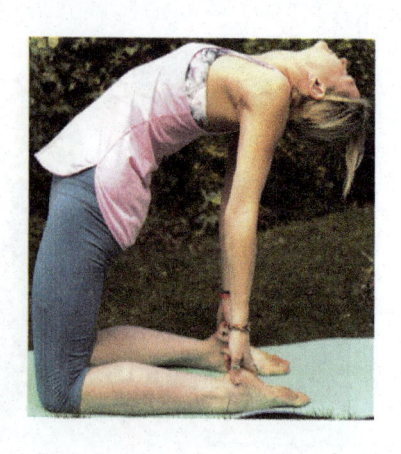

CAMEL POSE OR USHTRASANA

This posture is one of the most powerful heart openers. This pose leads to dramatic emotional releases. Do not be surprised if you are either sobbing or laughing during this backbend. This posture improves circulation in the brain and increases memory, concentration and reduces depression and stress.

STEP BY STEP

Do not practice this pose if you are currently experiencing high or low blood pressure, insomnia, or a migraine. Also avoid this pose if you have a lower back or neck injury. Always work within your own range of limits and abilities. If you have any medical concerns, talk with your doctor before practicing yoga.

Begin by kneeling upright with your knees hip-distance apart. Rotate your thighs inward and press your shins and the tops of your feet into the floor. Do not squeeze your buttocks.

Rest your hands on the back of your pelvis, with your fingers pointing to the floor. Lengthen your tailbone down toward the floor and widen the back of your pelvis.

Lean back, with your chin slightly tucked toward your chest.

Beginners can stay here, keeping their hands on their back pelvis.

If you are comfortable here, you can take the pose even deeper. Reach back and hold onto each heel. Your palms should rest on your heels with your fingers pointing toward your toes and your thumbs holding the outside of each foot.

Keep your thighs perpendicular to the floor, with your hips directly over your knees. If it is difficult to grasp your heels without feeling compression in your lower back, tuck your toes to elevate your heels. You can also rest your hands on yoga blocks placed to the outside of each foot.

Lift up through your pelvis, keeping your lower spine long. Turn your arms outward without squeezing your shoulder blades. Keep your head in a neutral position, or allow it to drop back without straining or crunching your neck.

Hold for 30-60 seconds. To release, bring your hands back to your front hips. Inhale, lead with your heart, and lift your torso by pushing your hips down toward the floor. Your head should come up last. Rest in Child's Pose (Balasana) or Corpse Pose (Savasana).

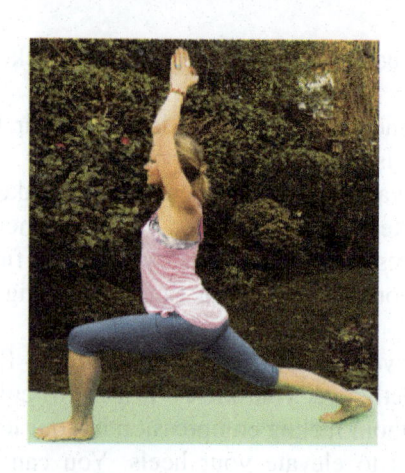

LUNGE POSE OR ANJANEYASANA

This posture strengthens the quadriceps and gluteus muscles, stretches the psoas and hips, relieves sciatica pain, expands your chest, lungs and shoulders, develops stamina and endurance in your thighs and improves your balance, concentration and core awareness. High lunge variations are designed to help ground the body. When it comes to bouncing back from relationships, getting grounded is the first and the most challenging thing to do.

Lunge variations are hip openers and once tension is released in the hips it helps the energy in the body become more stable.

STEP BY STEP

Do not practice Crescent Lunge if you are currently experiencing high blood pressure or heart problems. Also, avoid this pose if you have a knee or spinal injury. Always work within your own range of limits and abilities. If you have any medical concerns, talk with your doctor before practicing yoga.

Begin in Downward Facing Dog (Adho Mukha Svanasana). With an exhalation, step your right foot forward between your hands. Bend your front knee to 90 degrees, aligning your knee directly over the heel of your front foot.

Your feet should be hip-width apart with both feet facing forward, and your front shin should be perpendicular to the floor. Come on to the ball of your back foot, lifting your heel and drawing it forward so it aligns directly over your back toes.

Lift your back leg strongly, drawing your knee and quadriceps up toward the ceiling. Straighten your back leg completely. With your back leg strong and active, gently draw your left hip forward as you press your right hip back, squaring your hips so they are parallel to the top edge of your mat. If it is too difficult to keep your back leg raised while keeping your toes on the mat, lower your knee to the floor and slide your leg back a few inches.

Untuck your back toes and rest the top of your back foot on the floor.

Inhale as you raise your torso to an upright position. Sweep your arms overhead. Draw your tailbone toward the floor. Spin your pinky fingers toward each other, opening your arms so your palms face each other. Gently tilt your head and gaze up at a space between your thumbs.

Make sure your front shin stays vertical. Widen your stance as needed to make sure that your knee does not move forward past your ankle. Tuck your tailbone under and engage the muscles of your abdomen to help stabilize your core. Extend up through the crown of your head, lengthening your upper body. Draw your shoulder blades firmly into your upper back. Draw your lower front ribs in and down toward your belly — do not let them poke forward. Hold for up to one minute. Release your hands back to the mat and step back into Downward Dog. Repeat on the other side.

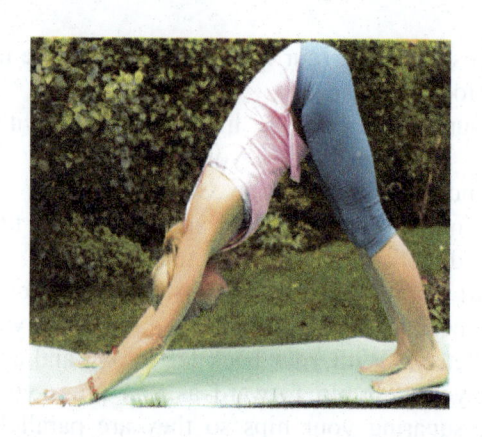

DOWNWARD DOG OR ADHO MUKHA SVANASANA

This posture elongates and releases tension from your spine, stretches your hamstrings, calves, arches, and hands, strengthens your arms, shoulders and back, improves the mobility of your digestive system and is a mild inversion that calms the onerous system and helps relieve stress.

STEP BY STEP

Come onto the floor on your hands and knees. Set your knees directly below your hips and your hands slightly forward of your shoulders. Spread your palms, index fingers parallel or slightly turned out, and turn your toes under.

Exhale and lift your knees away from the floor. At first keep the knees slightly bent and the heels lifted away from the floor. Lengthen your tailbone away from the back of your pelvis and press it lightly toward the pubis.

Against this resistance, lift the sitting bones toward the ceiling, and from your inner ankles draw the inner legs up into the groins. Then with an exhalation, push your top thighs back and stretch your heels onto or down toward the floor. Straighten your knees but be sure not to lock them. Firm the outer thighs and roll the upper thighs inward slightly. Narrow the front of the pelvis. Firm the outer arms and press the bases of the index fingers actively into the floor.

From these two points lift along your inner arms from the wrists to the tops of the shoulders. Firm your shoulder blades against your back, then widen them and draw them toward the tailbone. Keep the head between the upper arms; don't let it hang.

Adho Mukha Svanasana is one of the poses in the traditional Sun Salutation sequence. It's also an excellent yoga asana all on its own. Stay in this pose anywhere from one to three minutes. Then bend your knees to the floor with an exhalation and rest in Child's Pose.

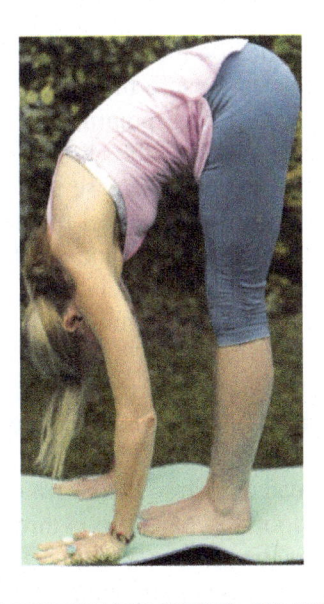

STANDING FORWARD BEND OR UTTANSANA

Forward bends are excellent for calming our nervous system. The posture provides a release of the upper body and soothes the mind through gentle inversion either when practiced on its own or between postures. This posture stretches your hips, hamstrings and calves, strengthens your thighs and knees, massages your internal organs and helps improve digestion and cleanses mucous from the lungs, relaxes your central nervous system and helps calm your mind, helps relieve stress, headaches, fatigue and insomnia; helps relieve symptoms of menopause and is therapeutic for osteoporosis.

As you stand in Mountain Pose (Tadasana), place your hands on your hips and inhale. As you exhale, soften your knees and fold slowly forward from your hips. Counterbalance your body weight by moving your tailbone and hips back slightly as the body leans forward. Keep your knees soft so your sit bones point up to the ceiling and your hip points roll forward into the upper thighs.

Rest your hands on the ground beside your feet or hold onto your elbows. Ensure that your feet are still parallel (second and middle toes pointing forward). Hollow out your belly and encourage the chest bone to float down to the top of your feet and increase the space between your pubis and your chest bone. Feel that the fold comes from your hip joint and not from rounding of your lower back.

If the hamstrings feel ease in this stetch, slowly extend your knees more while pushing your sit bones up to the ceiling.

Root into the heels as you slightly turn the top of the thighs inwards. This inwards rotation of your thighs aligns and isolates more of the inner hamstring lines.

Let your head dangle so the crown of your head reaches down to the floor so your gaze is through the legs. Hold for several slow breaths.

To exit, contract your abdominal and core muscles.

As you inhale, place your hands on your hips, soften your knees, and reach your chest far forward. Rise up from your hips keeping your back long. Keep the length between the pubis and chest bone. Continue to lengthen your torso as you come up to standing.

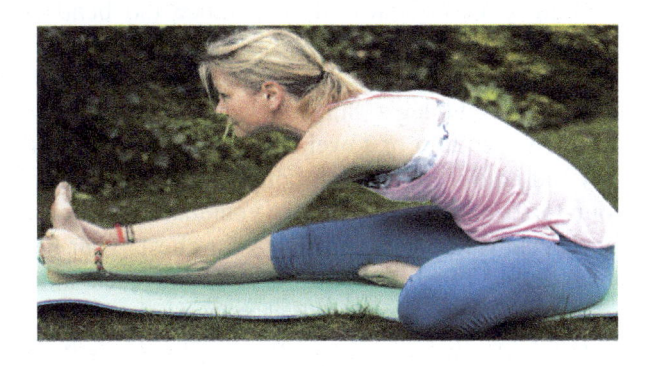

HEAD TO KNEE POSE OR JANU SIRSASANA

This posture stretches your spine, back muscles, hamstrings and groin, massages and stimulates your internal organs like the liver and kidneys, improves digestion and helps heal gastric ailments. It also calms the mind and central nervous system.

STEP BY STEP

Avoid practicing this pose if you are currently suffering from asthma or diarrhoea. Students with back or knee injuries should only practice this pose with the guidance of an experienced and knowledgeable teacher.

Always work within your own range of limits and abilities. If you have any medical concerns, talk with your doctor before practicing yoga.

Sit on the edge of a firm blanket, with your legs extended in front of you in Staff Pose (Dandasana). Bring the sole of your left foot to the inside of your right thigh. Align the centre of your torso with your right leg (a mild twist).

Keeping your spine long, exhale as you hinge forward from the hips to fold over your right leg. Imagine your torso coming to rest on your right thigh, rather than reaching your nose toward your knee (so bend at your waist).

Draw your right thigh down and flex your foot. Hold onto your right leg's shin, ankle, or foot. You can also wrap a yoga strap or towel around the sole of your right foot and hold it firmly with both hands. Keep the front of your torso long; do not round your back. Let your belly touch your thigh first, and then your chest. Your head and nose should touch your leg last. With each inhalation, lengthen the front torso. With each exhalation, fold deeper.

Hold for 30 seconds. To release the pose, draw your tailbone toward the floor as you inhale and lift your torso. Extend your left leg. Repeat the pose on the opposite side.

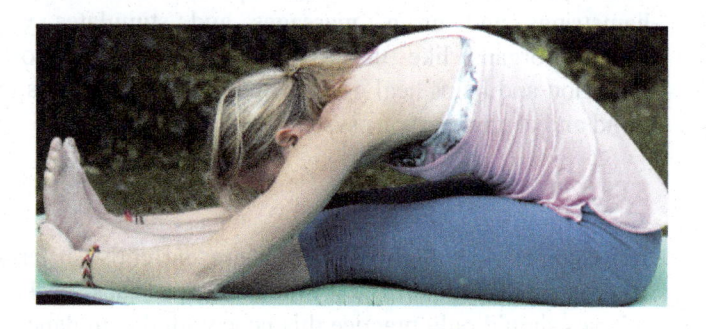

SEATED FORWARD BEND OR PASCHIMOTTANASANA

This asana stretches the hamstring, spine and lower back, calms the mind and relieves stress and anxiety, improves digestion, relieves symptoms of PMS and menopause, reduces fatigue and stimulates the liver, kidneys, ovaries, and uterus. Forward and backbends are great for removing anger, betrayal and all other negative emotions that cause spinal tension. This pose also helps increase awareness by releasing energies that cloud clear thought.

STEP BY STEP

Begin in a seated position with legs extended long and together and arms relaxed on either side. Take a big inhalation. On the exhalation, fall forward, pulling navel to spine and extending hands toward feet as much or as little as feels good on the legs and lower back. Allow the head to relax down toward the legs. (If hamstrings are tight, soften knees.) Breath here for as long as it feels good.

When you are ready to come out, one vertebra at a time, roll up and then onto back, keeping soft knees.

INSOMNIA/SELF OBSESSED

If the mind is still active when you lie down to sleep, it is almost impossible to fall asleep, no matter how tired you are. Our sympathetic nervous system is our 'get up and go' call and very often, in the stressed daily lives that we lead, it is still active when we lie down to get some rest. If you regularly suffer from insomnia it is essential that you calm the mind and activate the parasympathetic nervous system before going to bed. Do the asanas before going to bed.

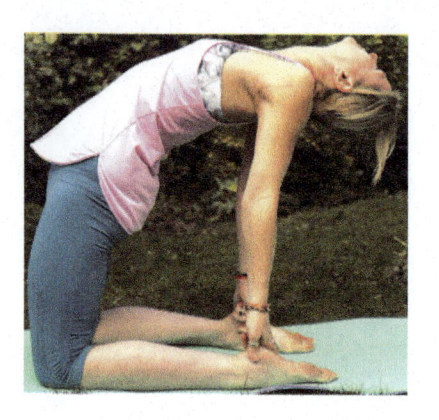

CAMEL POSE OR USHTRASANA

This posture is one of the most powerful heart openers. This pose leads to dramatic emotional releases. Do not be surprised if you are either sobbing or laughing during this backbend. This posture improves circulation in the brain and increases memory, concentration and reduces depression and stress.

STEP BY STEP

Do not practice this pose if you are currently experiencing high or low blood pressure, insomnia, or a migraine. Also avoid this pose if you have a lower back or neck injury.

Always work within your own range of limits and abilities. If you have any medical concerns, talk with your doctor before practicing yoga.

Begin by kneeling upright with your knees hip-distance apart. Rotate your thighs inward and press your shins and the tops of your feet into the floor. Do not squeeze your buttocks.

Rest your hands on the back of your pelvis, with your fingers pointing to the floor. Lengthen your tailbone down toward the floor and widen the back of your pelvis.

Lean back, with your chin slightly tucked toward your chest.

Beginners can stay here, keeping their hands on their back pelvis. If you are comfortable here, you can take the pose even deeper. Reach back and hold onto each heel. Your palms should rest on your heels with your fingers pointing toward your toes and your thumbs holding the outside of each foot.

Keep your thighs perpendicular to the floor, with your hips directly over your knees. If it is difficult to grasp your heels without feeling compression in your lower back, tuck your toes to elevate your heels. You can also rest your hands on yoga blocks placed to the outside of each foot.

Lift up through your pelvis, keeping your lower spine long. Turn your arms outward without squeezing your shoulder blades. Keep your head in a neutral position, or allow it to drop back without straining or crunching your neck.

Hold for 30-60 seconds. To release, bring your hands back to your front hips. Inhale, lead with your heart, and lift your torso by pushing your hips down toward the floor. Your head should come up last. Rest in Child's Pose (Balasana) or Corpse Pose (Savasana).

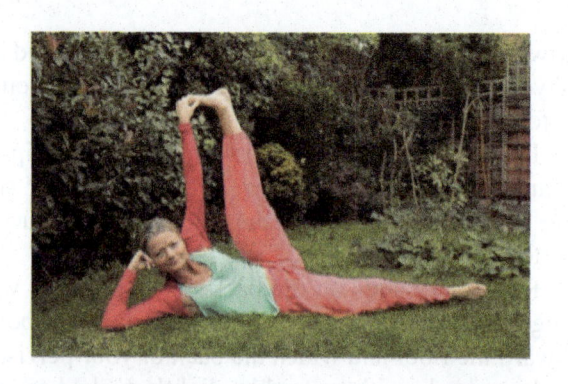

HAND TO FOOT POSE OR ANANTASANA

If you are unable to straighten your leg holding your toe, use a strap as an aid. Never try to force yourself into a position – remember that your body will place its own natural limitations on you.

STEP BY STEP

It begins rather simply. Lie on your side on your yoga mat. The goal is to line up your entire body flush with the edge of the mat.

Start with your bottom heel (keep your foot flexed) and then continue along the line of your leg. Line up your hip with your heel and then prop yourself up on your bottom elbow with your head in your hand.

Gently corset your ribs together so that the upper back stays along the edge of the mat. Adjust the angle of your bottom elbow to be in line with the mat.

You can keep your top foot and hand on the ground in front of you for balance. Look over your shoulder to make sure everything is straight and ready to go.

Once your body is in a long straight line, bend your top knee and place the sole of that foot in front of your bottom thigh.

Adjust your foot so that the toes and knee cap point toward your flexed base foot. Bring the pinky edge of your bent knee foot flush with your inner thigh.

Place your top hand to the inside of the top thigh and gently press back to open your hips and encourage external rotation. There is a tendency to pitch the lower back and puff the ribs. Counteract this by zippering your tailbone toward your flexed foot and drawing your front ribs in as if you've just tightened a corset around your ribcage.

Keep the action of your tailbone and ribcage as you hook your top leg big toe with your top hand. Before you extend your top leg, reaffirm the flex of the base foot and the engagement of the base leg. This leg will be your anchor to prevent you from falling. Slowly extend your top leg toward a straight position, keeping the top shoulder in the socket.

Externally rotate the top leg, taking the heel forward and toes back. Here's where the dance begins; don't panic if your body wobbles, this is normal. Just keep the intention of the anchored base leg, long tailbone and corseted ribcage.

Relax your gaze and head on your hand. Try to go for a solid eight breaths or longer if you're feeling inspired. Switch sides.

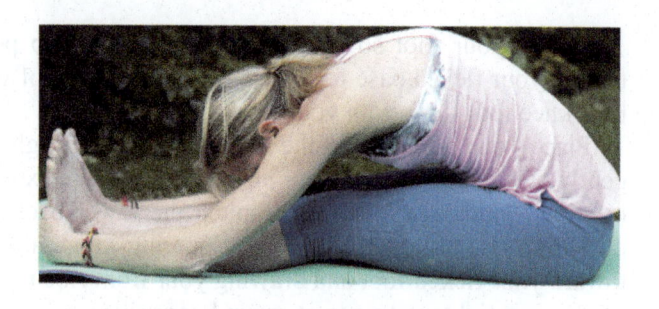

SEATED FORWARD BEND OR PASCHIMOTTANASANA

This asana stretches the hamstring, spine and lower back, calms the mind and relieves stress and anxiety, improves digestion, relieves symptoms of PMS and menopause, reduces fatigue and stimulates the liver, kidneys, ovaries, and uterus. Forward and backbends are great for removing anger, betrayal and all other negative emotions that cause spinal tension. This pose also helps increase awareness by releasing energies that cloud clear thought.

STEP BY STEP

Begin in a seated position with legs extended long and together and arms relaxed on either side. Take a big inhalation. On the exhalation, fall forward, pulling navel to spine and extending hands toward feet as much or as little as feels good on legs and lower back. Allow head to relax down toward legs. (If hamstrings are tight, soften knees.) Breath here for as long as it feels good.

When you are ready to come out, roll out one vertebra at a time.

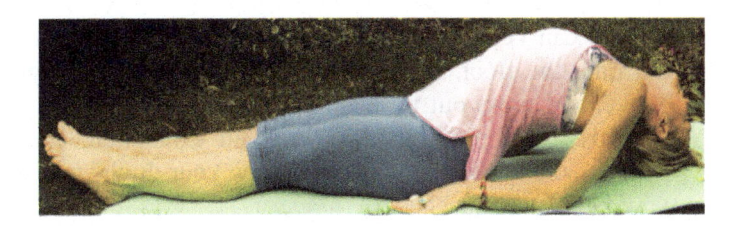

FISH POSE OR MATSYASANA

This particular posture is usually practiced following the Shoulder Stand as a counter-balance. After turning your world upside down, it's now time to focus on expanding and opening the heart and lung area. Fear often settles in this area, creating a kind of static that keeps us from being able to clearly hear our loving inner voice.

As your body weight rests on your legs, buttocks, forearms and the crown of the head, lift the rib cage and upper chest area as high as it will go upward. Create an opening directly from your heart...

STEP BY STEP

Lie on your back on the floor with your knees bent, feet on the floor. Inhale, lift your pelvis slightly off the floor, and slide your hands, palms down, below your buttocks. Then rest your buttocks on the backs of your hands (and don't lift them off your hands as you perform this pose). Be sure to tuck your forearms and elbows up close to the sides of your torso. Inhale and press your forearms and elbows firmly against the floor. Next, press your scapulas into your back and, with an inhalation, lift your upper torso and head away from the floor. Then release your head back onto the floor. Depending on how high you arch your back and lift your chest, either the back of your head or its crown will rest on the floor. There should be a minimal amount of weight on your head to avoid crunching your neck.

You can keep your knees bent or straighten your legs out onto the floor. If you do the latter, keep your thighs active, and press out through the heels. Stay for 15 to 30 seconds, breathing smoothly. With an exhalation, lower your torso and head to the floor. Draw your thighs up into your belly and squeeze.

DEPRESSION

Any posture that lifts the spirits – shoulder stands and plough postures are particularly good. As are back bends and forward bends. Twists release tension so a combination of postures is good. Linked to the crown chakra, meditation, Savasana, forward folds and shoulder stands are particularly good. Here are some suggested postures.

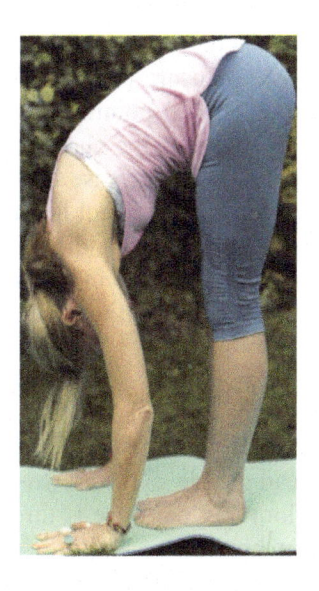

STANDING FORWARD BEND OR UTTANASANA

Forward bends are excellent for calming our nervous system. The posture provides a release of the upper body and soothes the mind through gentle inversion either when practiced on its own or between postures. This posture stretches your hips, hamstrings and calves, strengthens your thighs and knees, massages your internal organs and helps improve digestion and cleanses mucous from the lungs, relaxes your central nervous system and helps calm your mind, helps relieve stress, headaches, fatigue and insomnia; helps relieve symptoms of menopause and is therapeutic for osteoporosis.

As you stand in Mountain Pose (Tadasana), place your hands on your hips and inhale. As you exhale, soften your knees and fold slowly forward from your hips. Counterbalance your body weight by moving your tailbone and hips back slightly as the body leans forward. Keep your knees soft so your sit bones point up to the ceiling and your hip points roll forward into the upper thighs.

Rest your hands on the ground beside your feet or hold onto your elbows. Ensure that your feet are still parallel (second and middle toes pointing forward). Hollow out your belly and encourage the chest bone to float down to the top of your feet and increase the space between your pubis and your chest bone. Feel that the fold comes from your hip joint and not from rounding of your lower back.

If the hamstrings feel ease in this stetch, slowly extend your knees more while pushing your sit bones up to the ceiling.

Root into the heels as you slightly turn the top of the thighs inwards. This inwards rotation of your thighs aligns and isolates more of the inner hamstring lines.

Let your head dangle so the crown of your head reaches down to the floor so your gaze is through the legs. Hold for several slow breaths.

To exit, contract your abdominal and core muscles.

As you inhale, place your hands on your hips, soften your knees, and reach your chest far forward. Rise up from your hips keeping your back long. Keep the length between the pubis and chest bone. Continue to lengthen your torso as you come up to standing.

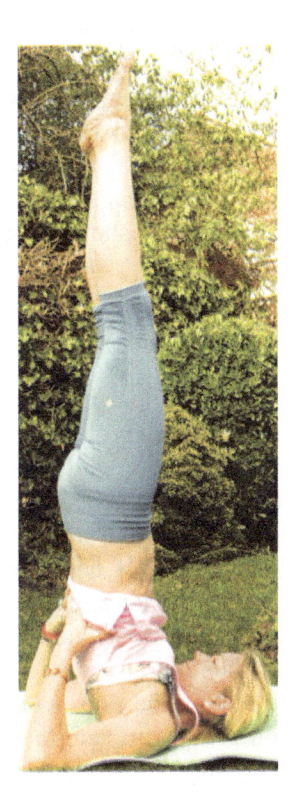

SHOULDER STAND OR SALAMBA SARVANGASANA

Balances the thyroid and hypothalamus glands, allowing for proper hormone production and reduces strain on the heart. Healthy blood can easily circulate around the neck and chest, and as a result, people with asthma, bronchitis and throat ailments may get relief. Helps you think differently about things – literally turning things on their head. Turns negatives into positives. This pose has a soothing effect on the parasympathetic nervous system. Therefore, those easily irritated, or prone to anger or nervous breakdowns can be stabilized and less reactive to life's circumstances. The change in gravitational pull on the body affects the abdominal organs so that the bowels move freely and constipation is relieved. Strengthens the upper body, legs and abdomen. The posture opens the chest and stretches the neck, shoulders and upper back muscles. What else? It decreases varicose veins, reduces wrinkles and helps you sleep. No wonder it's called the Queen of poses. Don't do shoulder stand in the first few days of your period.

STEP BY STEP

Begin in a seated position with legs extended long and together and arms relaxed on either side. Take a big inhalation. On the exhalation, fall forward, pulling navel to spine and extending hands toward feet as much or as little as feels good on the legs and lower back. Allow head to relax down toward legs. (If hamstrings are tight, soften knees.) Breath here for as long as it feels good.

When you are ready to come out, one vertebra at a time, roll up and then onto back, keeping soft knees. Bend knees and place feet on the floor with arms on either side. Soften knees and press arms into the ground to reach feet up toward the ceiling. Breath here for as long as it is comfortable.

When you feel comfortable, allow feet to fall back behind you an amount that feels good on your neck.

Reach feet to the ground for plough pose. Clasp hands together on the ground and wiggle shoulders underneath you one at a time. Press firmly into arms, reach through heels, and breath here for at least three deep breaths.

From plough or modified plough, place hands on lower back for support and try to keep elbows about shoulder-width apart. Soften legs and allow knees to rest on forehead in an egg shape. Breath here for as long as it is comfortable.

When you feel steady, reach feet toward ceiling one at a time, lengthening legs when you feel comfortable. Breath here for at least three deep breaths. To come down, slowly soften knees toward forehead, come back to plough, and slowly lower back to mat one vertebra at a time.

Fish is a great counterpart to shoulder stand and can be an effective way to relieve neck and back pain, improve circulation, and open your chest muscles.

Place hands and palms underneath butt and hips. Keep elbows as close together as possible and fingertips facing forward with forearms parallel to each other on the ground. Bend elbows and lean onto forearms, pressing them into the floor. Lift chest up toward the ceiling so that back is arched. Bring elbows toward each other until they're about shoulder-width apart. Allow head to relax down toward the ground until it touches the mat. Breath here for at least three deep breaths. When ready, come out of this slowly and lie on your back for a few breaths to enjoy how great you feel.

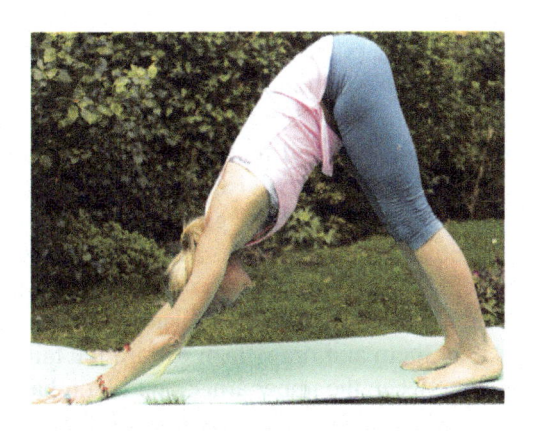

DOWNWARD FACING DOG OR ADHO MUKHA SVANASANA

Like the shoulder stand, this is an excellent cure all posture. Practice this posture and you gain stronger hands, wrists, lower back, hamstrings, calves and Achilles tendon. It also helps with back pain by strengthening the entire back and shoulder girdle, elongating the shoulders and shoulder blade area. Decreases tension and headaches by elongating the cervical spine and neck and relaxing the head. Deepens respiration, decreases anxiety, increases full-body circulation.

STEP BY STEP

Come onto the floor on your hands and knees. Set your knees directly below your hips and your hands slightly forward of your shoulders. Spread your palms, index fingers parallel or slightly turned out, and turn your toes under. Exhale and lift your knees away from the floor. At first keep the knees slightly bent and the heels lifted away from the floor. Lengthen your tailbone away from the back of your pelvis and press it lightly toward the pubis. Against this resistance, lift the sitting bones toward the ceiling, and from your inner ankles draw the inner legs up into the groins.

Then with an exhalation, push your top thighs back and stretch your heels onto or down toward the floor. Straighten your knees but be sure not to lock them. Firm the outer thighs and roll the upper thighs inward slightly. Narrow the front of the pelvis.

Firm the outer arms and press the bases of the index fingers actively into the floor. From these two points lift along your inner arms from the wrists to the tops of the shoulders. Firm your shoulder blades against your back, then widen them and draw them toward the tailbone. Keep the head between the upper arms; don't let it hang.

Adho Mukha Svanasana is one of the poses in the traditional Sun Salutation sequence. It's also an excellent yoga asana all on its own. Stay in this pose anywhere from one to three minutes. Then bend your knees to the floor with an exhalation and rest in Child's Pose.

PMS (PRE MENSTRUAL SYNDROME)

How many symptoms does this 'infliction' include? It seem endless but let's start with irritability, moodiness, anger, fear, tearfulness…… Try the following:

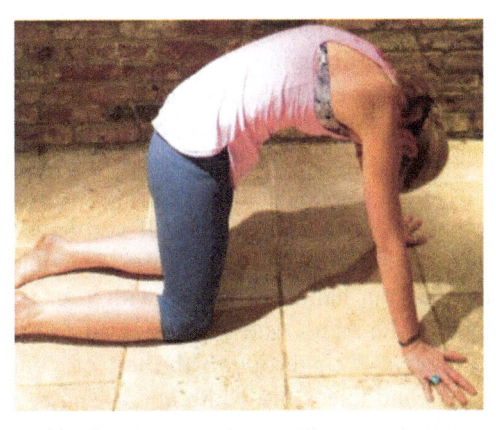

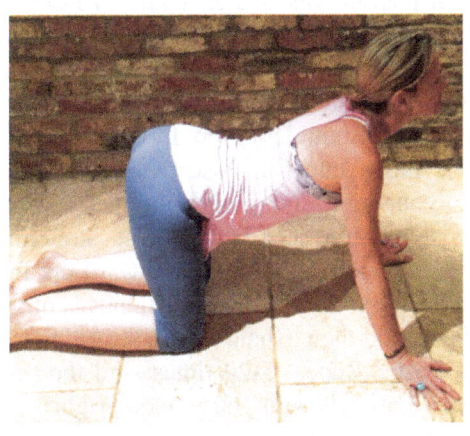

**CAT AND COW POSE/MARJARIASANA
AND BITILASANA**

This posture tones and relaxes the spine and abdomen and improves posture and balance. Strengthens and stretches the spine and neck. Stretches the hips, abdomen and back. Increases coordination. Massages and stimulates organs in the belly, like the kidneys and adrenal glands. Creates emotional balance. Relieves stress and calms the mind.

STEP BY STEP

Those with neck injuries should keep the head in line with the torso, not dropping it forward or back. Pregnant women and those with back injuries should only perform Cow Pose, bringing the spine back to neutral between poses — do not let the belly drop between repetitions, as this can strain the lower back. Always work within your own range of limits and abilities. If you have any medical concerns, talk with your doctor before practicing yoga.

Start on your hands and knees with your wrists directly under your shoulders, and your knees directly under your hips. Point your fingertips to the top of your mat. Place your shins and knees hip-width apart. Centre your head in a neutral position and soften your gaze downward. Begin by moving into Cow Pose. Inhale as you drop your belly towards the mat. Lift your chin and chest, and gaze up toward the ceiling. Broaden across your shoulder blades and draw your shoulders away from your ears.

Next, move into Cat Pose. As you exhale, draw your belly to your spine and round your back toward the ceiling. The pose should look like a cat stretching its back. Release the crown of your head toward the floor, but don't force your chin to your chest. Inhale, coming back into Cow Pose, and then exhale as you return to

Cat Pose. Repeat 5-20 times, and then rest by sitting back on your heels with your torso upright.

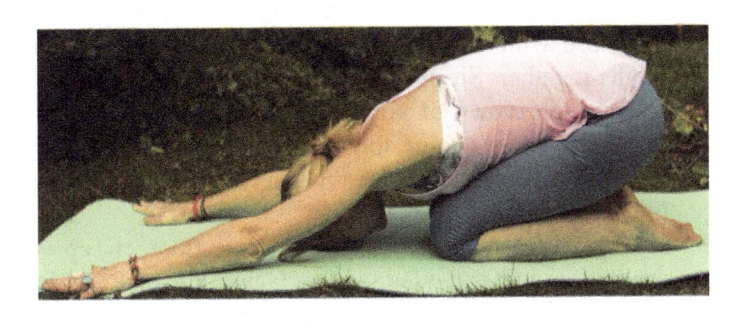

CHILD POSE OR BALASANA

Calms the nervous system and soothes the back. Releases tension in the back, shoulders and chest. Recommended if you have dizziness or fatigue. Helps alleviate stress and anxiety. Flexes the body's internal organs and keeps them supple. It lengthens and stretches the spine. Relieves neck and lower back pain when performed with the head and torso supported. It gently stretches the hips, thighs and ankles. Normalizes circulation throughout the body. It stretches muscles, tendons and ligaments in the knee. Calms the mind and body. Encourages strong and steady breathing

STEP BY STEP

Do not practice Child's Pose if you have a current or recent knee injury. Women who are pregnant should only practice a wide-legged variation of the pose — do not press the belly on top of the thighs. Always work within your own range of limits and abilities. If you have any medical concerns, talk with your doctor before practicing yoga.

Begin on your hands and knees. Centre your breath, and begin to let your thoughts slow down. Turn your awareness inward. Spread your knees wide apart while keeping your big toes touching. Rest your buttocks on your heels.

Those with very tight hips can keep their knees and thighs together. Sit up straight and lengthen your spine up through the crown of your head. On an exhalation, bow forward, draping your torso between your thighs. Your heart and chest should rest between or on top of your thighs.

Allow your forehead to come to the floor. Keep your arms long and extended, palms facing down. Press back slightly with your hands to keep your buttocks in contact with your heels. Lengthen from your hips to your armpits, and then extend even further through your fingertips. For deeper relaxation, bring your arms back to rest alongside your thighs with your palms facing up.

Completely relax your elbows. Let your upper back broaden. Soften and relax your lower back. Allow all tension in your shoulders, arms, and neck to drain away.

Keep your gaze drawn inward with your eyes closed. Hold for up to a minute or longer, breathing softly. To release the pose, gently use your hands to walk your torso upright to sit back on your heels.

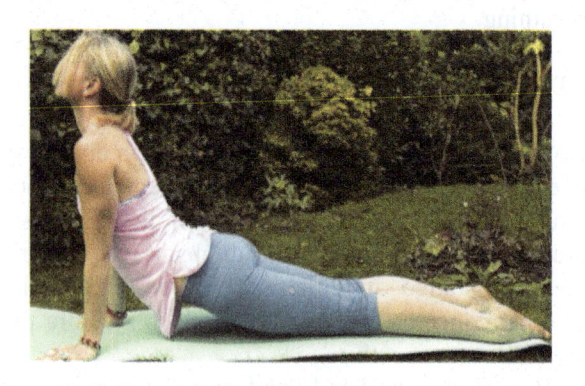

COBRA POSE OR BHUJANGASANA

Great for blood circulation and relaxing the back. Stretches muscles in the shoulders, chest and abdominals.

Decreases stiffness of the lower back. Strengthens the arms and shoulders. Increases flexibility. Improves menstrual irregularities. Elevates mood. Firms and tones the buttocks. Invigorates the heart. Stimulates organs in the abdomen, like the kidneys. Relieves stress and fatigue. Opens the chest and helps to clear the passages of the heart and lungs. Improves circulation of blood and oxygen, especially throughout the spinal and pelvic regions. Improves digestion. Strengthens the spine. Soothes sciatica. Helps to ease symptoms of asthma.

STEP BY STEP

Lie prone on the floor. Stretch your legs back, tops of the feet on the floor. Spread your hands on the floor under your shoulders. Hug the elbows back into your body.

Press the tops of the feet and thighs and the pubis firmly into the floor.

On an inhalation, begin to straighten the arms to lift the chest off the floor, going only to the height at which you can maintain a connection through your pubis to your legs. Press the tailbone toward the pubis and lift the pubis toward the navel. Narrow the hip points. Firm but don't harden the buttocks.

Firm the shoulder blades against the back, puffing the side ribs forward. Lift through the top of the sternum but avoid pushing the front ribs forward, which only hardens the lower back. Distribute the backbend evenly throughout the entire spine.

Hold the pose anywhere from 15 to 30 seconds, breathing easily. Release back to the floor with an exhalation.

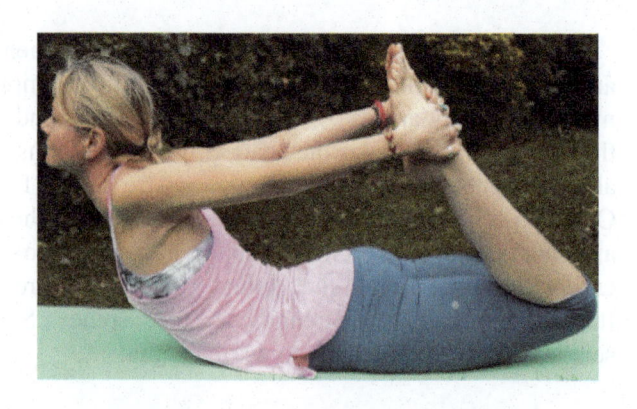

BOW POSE OR DHANURASANA

This is ideal for menstrual discomfort and removes fatigue. Strengthens the back and abdominal muscles. Stimulates the reproductive organs. Opens up the chest, neck and shoulders. Tones the leg and arm muscles

Helps people with renal (kidney) disorders. Do not practice Bow Pose (Dhanurasana) if you have high or low blood pressure, hernia, neck injury, pain in the lower back, headache, migraine or recent abdominal surgery. Ladies should avoid practicing this yoga pose during pregnancy.

STEP BY STEP

Do not practice this pose if you are currently experiencing high or low blood pressure, headaches, diarrhoea, or heart problems. Also avoid this pose if you have a back injury or carpal tunnel syndrome.

Upward Bow requires a great deal of strength and flexibility to be performed correctly. It is very easy to injure yourself if you attempt to move into it too soon, if you do not yet have the strength or flexibility to do the pose in correct alignment.

Do not practice this pose if you are currently experiencing high or low blood pressure, migraines, or insomnia. Also avoid this pose if you are pregnant, or if you have a low-back or neck injury.

Always work within your own range of limits and abilities. If you have any medical concerns, talk with your doctor before practicing yoga.

Begin by lying flat on your stomach with your chin on the mat and your hands resting at your sides.

On an exhalation, bend your knees. Bring your heels as close as you can to your buttocks, keeping your knees hip-distance apart.

Reach back with both hands and hold onto your outer ankles. On an inhalation, lift your heels up toward the ceiling, drawing your thighs up and off the mat. Your head, chest, and upper torso will also lift off the mat.

Draw your tailbone down firmly into the floor, while you simultaneously lift your heels and thighs even higher. Lift your chest and press your shoulder blades firmly into your upper back. Draw your shoulders away from your ears. Gaze forward and breath softly. Your breath will become shallow, but do not hold your breath. Hold for up to 30 seconds. To release, exhale and gently lower your thighs to the mat. Slowly release your legs and feet to the floor. Place your right ear on the mat and relax your arms at your sides for a few breaths.

Repeat the pose for the same amount of time, then rest with your left ear on the mat.

LONELINESS/PANIC ATTACKS

Feeling you are alone can lead to depression. But you are never alone. The feeling of loneliness is nothing to do with what is happening around you, it is to do with what is happening within you. Closely linked to feelings of self-esteem, any posture that improves self-esteem (which is linked to the solar plexus chakra (Manipura chakra) will help you. All twisting postures are good and standing forward folds as well as sun salutations. Here are some suggested postures. Anxiety also strikes when you are going through menopause or midlife crisis (which may occur at any time actually) so if you are at that time in life, try out these postures, it will help with the anxiety you may feel before you go to bed and when you wake up.

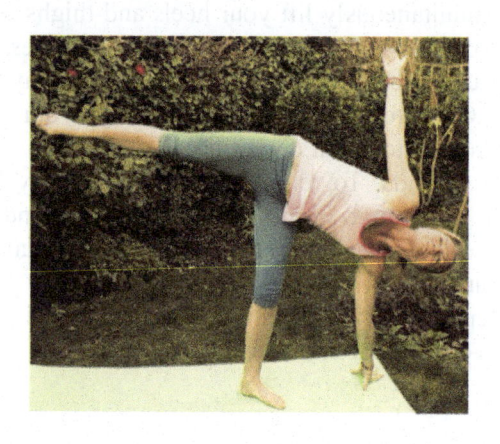

HALF MOON POSE OR ARDHA CHANDRASANA

This asana quiets the mind yet brings awareness. Half Moon is a balancing posture with one leg raised 90 degrees and one hand on the floor or on a block. Balancing poses take our attention from our mind and into our body, expands your chest and shoulders, increases the mobility of your hip joints, increases neck mobility, lengthens your spinal muscles, strengthens and tones the muscles of your thighs and calves, stretches your hamstrings and groin muscles and increases proprioception (the sense of position in space) of the feet and ankles.

STEP BY STEP

Do not practice Half Moon Pose if you have low blood pressure or are currently experiencing headaches, insomnia, or diarrhoea. Those with neck injuries should not turn their heads to face the top hand, but should continue looking straight ahead. Always work within your own range of limits and abilities. If you have any medical concerns, talk with your doctor before practicing yoga.

Begin by standing at the top of your mat. Turn to the left and step your feet wide apart. Extend your arms out to the sides at shoulder-height. Your feet should be as far apart as your wrists. Rotate your right (front) foot 90 degrees, so your front foot's toes point to the top of the mat. Turn your left foot's toes slightly in. Align your front heel with the arch of your back foot. Reach through your right hand in the same direction that your right foot is pointed. Shift your left hip back, and then fold sideways at the hip. Rest your right hand on your outer right shin or ankle. If you are more flexible, place your fingertips on the floor. You can also place your hand on a block.

Align your shoulders so your left shoulder is directly above your right shoulder. Gently turn your head to gaze at your left thumb. Bring your left hand to rest on your left hip. Turn your head to look at the floor. Then bend your right knee and step your left foot 6-12 inches closer to your right foot. Place your right hand's fingertips on the floor in front of your right foot. Press firmly into your right hand and foot. Straighten your right leg while simultaneously lifting your left leg. Work toward bringing your left leg parallel to the floor, or even higher than your hips. Reach actively through your left heel. Do not lock your right leg's knee. Keep your right foot's toes and kneecap facing in the direction of your head.

Stack your top hip directly over your bottom hip, and open your torso to the left. Then extend your left arm and point your fingertips directly toward the sky. If you can balance comfortably there, turn your head and gaze at your left thumb. Draw your shoulder blades firmly into your back. Lengthen your tailbone toward your left heel. Hold for up to one minute. To release, lower your left leg as you exhale. Return to Extended Triangle Pose. Inhale and press firmly through your left heel as you lift your torso. Lower your arms. Turn to the left, reversing the position of your feet, and repeat for the same length of time on the opposite side.

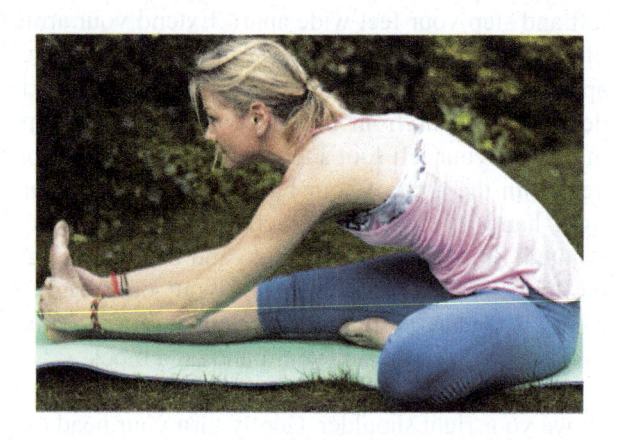

HEAD TO KNEE POSE OR JANU SIRSASANA

This posture stretches your spine, back muscles, hamstrings and groin, massages and stimulates your internal organs like the liver and kidneys, improves digestion and helps heal gastric ailments. It also calms the mind and central nervous system.

STEP BY STEP

Avoid practicing this pose if you are currently suffering from asthma or diarrhoea. Students with back or knee injuries should only practice this pose with the guidance of an experienced and knowledgeable teacher.

Always work within your own range of limits and abilities. If you have any medical concerns, talk with your doctor before practicing yoga.

Sit on the edge of a firm blanket, with your legs extended in front of you in Staff Pose (Dandasana). Bring the sole of your left foot to the inside of your right thigh.

Align the centre of your torso with your right leg (a mild twist). Keeping your spine long, exhale as you hinge forward from the hips to fold over your right leg. Imagine your torso coming to rest on your right thigh, rather than reaching your nose toward your knee (so bend at your waist). Draw your right thigh down and flex your foot. Hold onto your right leg's shin, ankle, or foot. You can also wrap a yoga strap or towel around the sole of your right foot and hold it firmly with both hands. Keep the front of your torso long; do not round your back.

Let your belly touch your thigh first, and then your chest. Your head and nose should touch your leg last. With each inhalation, lengthen the front torso. With each exhalation, fold deeper. Hold for 30 seconds. To release the pose, draw your tailbone toward the floor as you inhale and lift your torso. Extend your left leg. Repeat the pose on the opposite side.

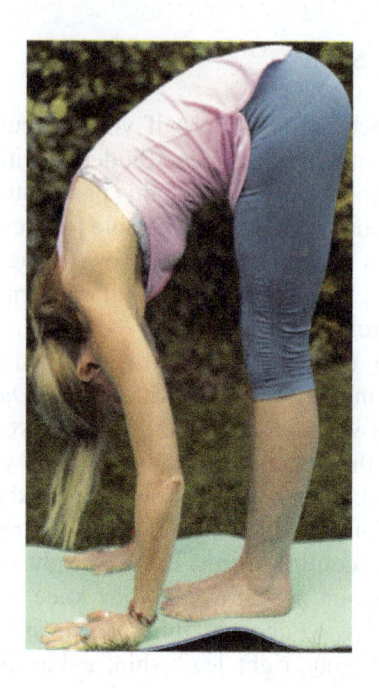

STANDING FORWARD BEND OR UTTANASANA

Forward bends are excellent for calming our nervous system. The posture provides a release of the upper body and soothes the mind through gentle inversion, either when practiced on its own or between postures. This posture stretches your hips, hamstrings and calves, strengthens your thighs and knees, massages your internal organs and helps improve digestion and cleanses mucus from the lungs, relaxes your central nervous system and helps calm your mind, helps relieve stress, headaches, fatigue and insomnia; helps relieve symptoms of menopause and is therapeutic for osteoporosis.

As you stand in Mountain Pose (Tadasana), place your hands on your hips and inhale. As you exhale, soften your knees and fold slowly forward from your hips. Counterbalance your body weight by moving your tailbone

and hips back slightly as the body leans forward. Keep your knees soft so your sit bones point up to the ceiling and your hip points roll forward into the upper thighs.

Rest your hands on the ground beside your feet or hold onto your elbows. Ensure that your feet are still parallel (second and middle toes pointing forward). Hollow out your belly and encourage the chest bone to float down to the top of your feet and increase the space between your pubis and your chest bone. Feel that the fold comes from your hip joint and not from rounding of your lower back.

If the hamstrings feel ease in this stetch, slowly extend your knees more while pushing your sit bones up to the ceiling.

Root into the heels as you slightly turn the top of the thighs inwards. This inwards rotation of your thighs aligns and isolates more of the inner hamstring lines.

Let your head dangle so the crown of your head reaches down to the floor so your gaze is through the legs. Hold for several slow breaths.

To exit, contract your abdominal and core muscles.

As you inhale, place your hands on your hips, soften your knees, and reach your chest far forward. Rise up from your hips keeping your back long. Keep the length between the pubis and chest bone. Continue to lengthen your torso as you come up to standing.

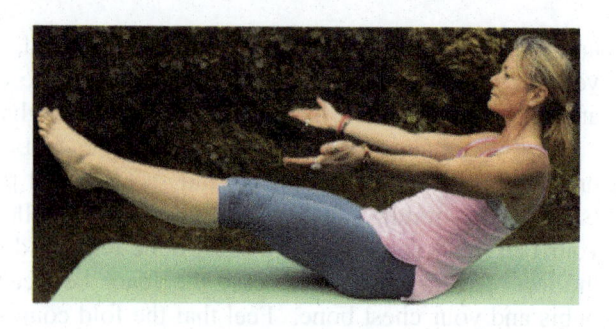

NAVASANA OR BOAT POSE

Strengthens the back and abdominal muscles, tones the legs and arm muscles and is useful for people with hernia.

STEP BY STEP

Sit on the floor with your legs straight in front of you. Press your hands on the floor a little behind your hips, fingers pointing toward the feet, and strengthen the arms. Lift through the top of the sternum and lean back slightly. As you do this make sure your back doesn't round; continue to lengthen the front of your torso between the pubis and top sternum. Sit on the "tripod" of your two sitting bones and tailbone.

Exhale and bend your knees, then lift your feet off the floor, so that the thighs are angled about 45-50 degrees relative to the floor.

Lengthen your tailbone into the floor and lift your pubis toward your navel. If possible, slowly straighten your knees, raising the tips of your toes slightly above the level of your eyes. If this isn't possible, remain with your knees bent, perhaps lifting the shins parallel to the floor.

Stretch your arms alongside the legs, parallel to each other and the floor. Spread the shoulder blades across your back and reach strongly out through the fingers. If this isn't possible, keep the hands on the floor beside your hips or hold on to the backs of your thighs.

While the lower belly should be firm, it shouldn't get hard and thick.

Try to keep the lower belly relatively flat. Press the heads of the thigh bones toward the floor to help anchor the pose and lift the top sternum. Breath easily. Tip the chin slightly toward the sternum so the base of the skull lifts lightly away from the back of the neck.

At first stay in the pose for 10-20 seconds. Gradually increase the time of your stay to one minute. Release the legs with an exhalation and sit upright on an inhalation.

GREED

Not knowing when enough is enough; any posture which focuses on improving acceptance and letting go is a good one for greed, also any posture which suppresses appetite. All back bends do this. Shoulder stand (Salamba Sarvangasana) is particularly good. Here are some suggested postures.

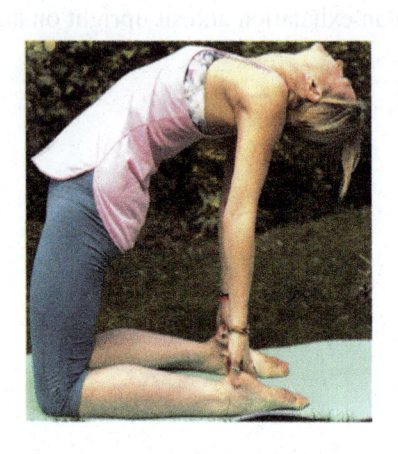

CAMEL POSE OR USHTRASANA

This posture is one of the most powerful heart openers. This pose leads to dramatic emotional releases. Do not be surprised if you are either sobbing or laughing during this backbend. This posture improves circulation in the brain and increases memory, concentration and reduces depression and stress.

STEP BY STEP

Do not practice this pose if you are currently experiencing high or low blood pressure, insomnia, or a migraine. Also avoid this pose if you have a lower back or neck injury. Always work within your own range of limits and abilities.

If you have any medical concerns, talk with your doctor before practicing yoga.

Begin by kneeling upright with your knees hip-distance apart. Rotate your thighs inward and press your shins and the tops of your feet into the floor. Do not squeeze your buttocks.

Rest your hands on the back of your pelvis, with your fingers pointing to the floor. Lengthen your tailbone down toward the floor and widen the back of your pelvis.

Lean back, with your chin slightly tucked toward your chest. Beginners can stay here, keeping their hands on their back pelvis.

If you are comfortable here, you can take the pose even deeper. Reach back and hold onto each heel. Your palms should rest on your heels with your fingers pointing toward your toes and your thumbs holding the outside of each foot.

Keep your thighs perpendicular to the floor, with your hips directly over your knees. If it is difficult to grasp your heels without feeling compression in your lower back, tuck your toes to elevate your heels. You can also rest your hands on yoga blocks placed to the outside of each foot.

Lift up through your pelvis, keeping your lower spine long. Turn your arms outward without squeezing your shoulder blades. Keep your head in a neutral position, or allow it to drop back without straining or crunching your neck.

Hold for 30-60 seconds. To release, bring your hands back to your front hips. Inhale, lead with your heart, and lift your torso by pushing your hips down toward the floor. Your head should come up last. Rest in Child's Pose (Balasana) or Corpse Pose (Savasana).

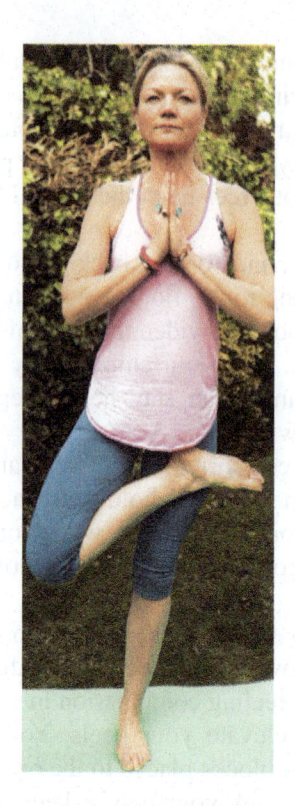

TREE POSE OR VRKSASANA

Improves focus and sense of balance. Supports a feeling of connection with the Earth and current environment. Starting in Mountain pose, begin to shift weight into left foot, bending right knee to bring your right foot and ankle to your calf or inner thigh of left leg. Focus eyes on the ground three to five feet in front of you. If you have a hard time balancing, rest one or both hands against a wall. Encourage both hips to be in a neutral position, parallel to the floor. Bring palms to touch at your heart's centre, interlacing middle, ring and pinkie fingers, leaving index fingers and thumbs extended. Press left foot firmly into the ground. Inhale and extend arms overhead, lengthening up. Hold for eight to ten diaphragmatic breaths, then on an exhalation return to Mountain pose and repeat on opposite side.

STEP BY STEP

Improves focus and sense of balance. Supports a feeling of connection with the Earth and current environment.

Starting in Mountain pose, begin to shift weight into left foot bending right knee to bring your right foot and ankle to your calf or inner thigh of left leg.

Focus eyes on the Earth three to five feet in front of you. If you have a hard time balancing, rest one or both hands against a wall. Encourage both hips to be in a neutral position, parallel to the floor.

Bring palms to touch at your heart's centre, interlacing middle, ring and pinkie fingers, leaving index fingers and thumbs extended. Press left foot firmly into the ground.

Inhale and extend arms overhead lengthening up. Hold for eight to 10 diaphragmatic breaths (see mountain pose), then on an exhalation return to mountain pose and repeat on opposite side.

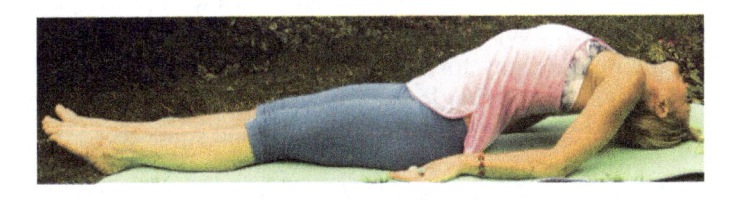

FISH POSE OR MATSYASANA

This particular posture is usually practiced following the Shoulder Stand as a counter-balance. After turning your world upside down, it's now time to focus on expanding and opening the heart and lung area. Fear often settles in this area, creating a kind of static that keeps us from being able to clearly hear our loving inner voice.

As your body weight rests on your legs, buttocks, forearms and the crown of the head, lift the rib cage and upper chest area as high as it will go upward. Create an opening directly from your heart...

STEP BY STEP

Lie on your back on the floor with your knees bent, feet on the floor. Inhale, lift your pelvis slightly off the floor, and slide your hands, palms down, below your buttocks. Then rest your buttocks on the backs of your hands (and don't lift them off your hands as you perform this pose). Be sure to tuck your forearms and elbows up close to the sides of your torso. Inhale and press your forearms and elbows firmly against the floor. Next press your scapulas into your back and, with an inhalation, lift your upper torso and head away from the floor.

Then release your head back onto the floor. Depending on how high you arch your back and lift your chest, either the back of your head or its crown will rest on the floor. There should be a minimal amount of weight on your head to avoid crunching your neck. You can keep your knees bent or straighten your legs out onto the floor. If you do the latter, keep your thighs active, and press out through the heels. Stay for 15 to 30 seconds, breathing smoothly. With an exhalation lower your torso and head to the floor. Draw your thighs up into your belly and squeeze.

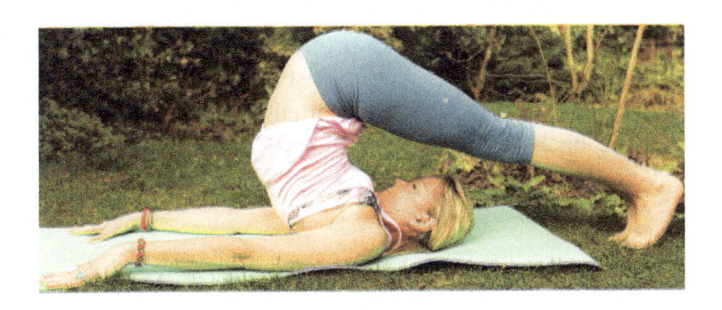

PLOUGH POSE OR HALASANA

This posture stretches the shoulders and improves the flexibility of your spine, calms your brain and nervous system and helps relieve stress and fatigue, improves digestion, massages and stimulates the thyroid gland, massages the abdominal organs and improves digestion, helps relieve the symptoms of menopause, and flushes mucous from your lungs.

STEP BY STEP

Begin in a seated position with legs extended long and together and arms relaxed on either side. Take a big inhale. On the exhale, fall forward, pulling navel to spine and extending hands toward feet as much or as little as feels good on the legs and lower back. Allow head to relax down toward legs. (If hamstrings are tight, soften knees.) Breath here for as long as it feels good.

When you are ready to come out, one vertebra at a time, roll up and then onto back, keeping soft knees. Bend knees and place feet on the floor with arms on either side. Soften knees and press arms into the ground to reach feet up toward the ceiling. Breath here for as long as is comfortable.

When you feel comfortable, allow feet to fall back behind you an amount that feels good on your neck.

Reach feet to the ground for plough pose. Clasp hands together on the ground and wiggle shoulders underneath you one at a time. Press firmly into arms, reach through heels, and breath here for at least three deep breaths.

To come down, slowly soften knees toward forehead, come back to plough, and slowly lower back to mat one vertebra at a time.

JEALOUSY/ENVY

The grass is not greener on the other side, it is just not on your side of the fence. When you realise this you will focus on what you have, be grateful and have an overwhelming sense of acceptance. When this happens you will be more contented and focus your energies and not on others. Don't give them your time or thought. All back bends and forward bends are good for this emotion, which has no upside, and balances, allowing you to concentrate only on the posture, breath and nothing else. Here are some suggested postures.

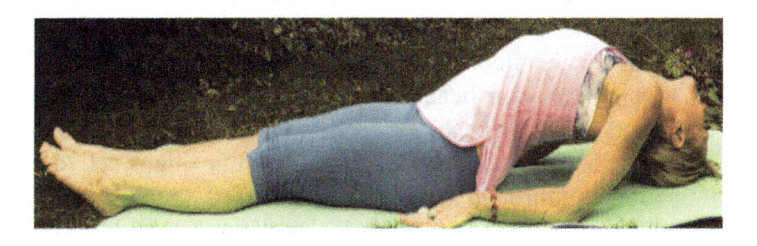

FISH POSE OR MATSYASANA

This particular posture is usually practiced following the Shoulder Stand, as a counter-balance. After turning your world upside down, it's now time to focus on expanding and opening the heart and lung area. Fear often settles in this area, creating a kind of static that keeps us from being able to clearly hear our loving inner voice. As your body weight rests on your legs, buttocks, forearms and the crown of the head, lift the rib cage and upper chest area as high as it will go upward. Create an opening directly from your heart...

STEP BY STEP

Lie on your back on the floor with your knees bent, feet on the floor. Inhale, lift your pelvis slightly off the floor, and slide your hands, palms down, below your buttocks. Then rest your buttocks on the backs of your hands (and don't lift them off your hands as you perform this pose). Be sure to tuck your forearms and elbows up close to the sides of your torso.

Inhale and press your forearms and elbows firmly against the floor. Next press your scapulas into your back and, with an inhalation, lift your upper torso and head away from the floor. Then release your head back onto the floor. Depending on how high you arch your back and lift your chest, either the back of your head or its crown will rest on the floor. There should be a minimal amount of weight on your head to avoid crunching your neck. You can keep your knees bent or straighten your legs out onto the floor. If you do the latter, keep your thighs active, and press out through the heels.

Stay for 15 to 30 seconds, breathing smoothly. With an exhalation lower your torso and head to the floor. Draw your thighs up into your belly and squeeze.

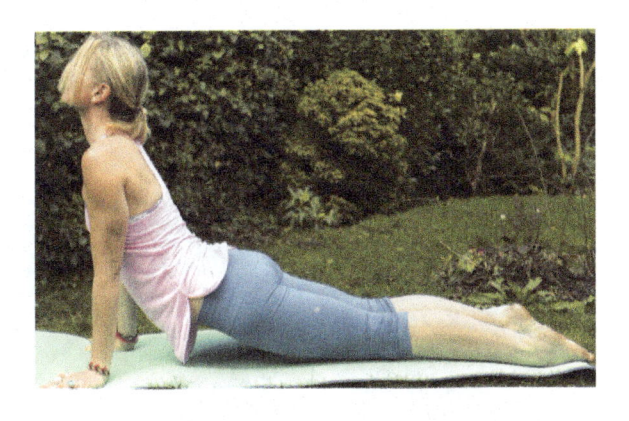

COBRA POSE OR BHUJANGASANA

This posture strengthens your back muscles and arms, increases the flexibility of your spine, stretches your chest, shoulders, lungs, and abdomen, and stretches and massages your internal organs and firms your buttocks.

STEP BY STEP

Lie prone on the floor. Stretch your legs back, tops of the feet on the floor. Spread your hands on the floor under your shoulders. Hug the elbows back into your body.

Press the tops of the feet and thighs and the pubis firmly into the floor.

On an inhalation, begin to straighten the arms to lift the chest off the floor, going only to the height at which you can maintain a connection through your pubis to your legs. Press the tailbone toward the pubis and lift the pubis toward the navel. Narrow the hip points. Firm but don't harden the buttocks.

Firm the shoulder blades against the back, puffing the side ribs forward. Lift through the top of the sternum but avoid pushing the front ribs forward, which only hardens the lower back. Distribute the backbend evenly throughout the entire spine.

Hold the pose anywhere from 15 to 30 seconds, breathing easily. Release back to the floor with an exhalation.

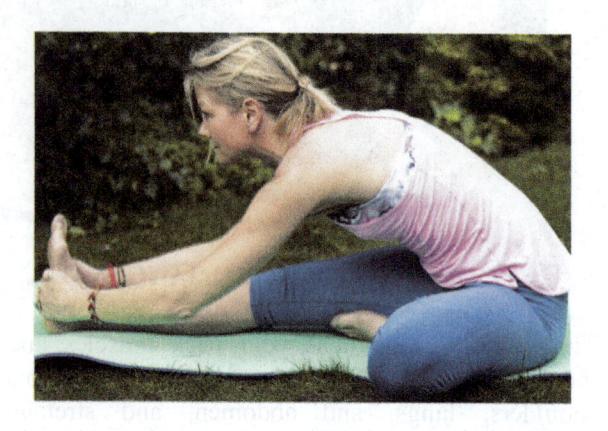

HEAD TO KNEE POSE OR JANU SIRSASANA

This posture stretches your spine, back muscles, hamstrings and groin, massages and stimulates your internal organs like the liver and kidneys, improves digestion and helps heal gastric ailments. It also calms the mind and central nervous system.

STEP BY STEP

Avoid practicing this pose if you are currently suffering from asthma or diarrhoea. Students with back or knee injuries should only practice this pose with the guidance of an experienced and knowledgeable teacher.

Always work within your own range of limits and abilities. If you have any medical concerns, talk with your doctor before practicing yoga.

Sit on the edge of a firm blanket, with your legs extended in front of you in Staff Pose (Dandasana). Bring the sole of your left foot to the inside of your right thigh. Align the centre of your torso with your right leg (a mild twist). Keeping your spine long, exhale as you hinge forward from the hips to fold over your right leg. Imagine your torso coming to rest on your right thigh, rather than reaching your nose toward your knee (so bend at your waist).

Draw your right thigh down and flex your foot. Hold onto your right leg's shin, ankle, or foot. You can also wrap a yoga strap or towel around the sole of your right foot and hold it firmly with both hands. Keep the front of your torso long; do not round your back.

Let your belly touch your thigh first, and then your chest. Your head and nose should touch your leg last. With each inhalation, lengthen the front torso. With each exhalation, fold deeper. Hold for 30 seconds. To release the pose, draw your tailbone toward the floor as you inhale and lift your torso. Extend your left leg. Repeat the pose on the opposite side.

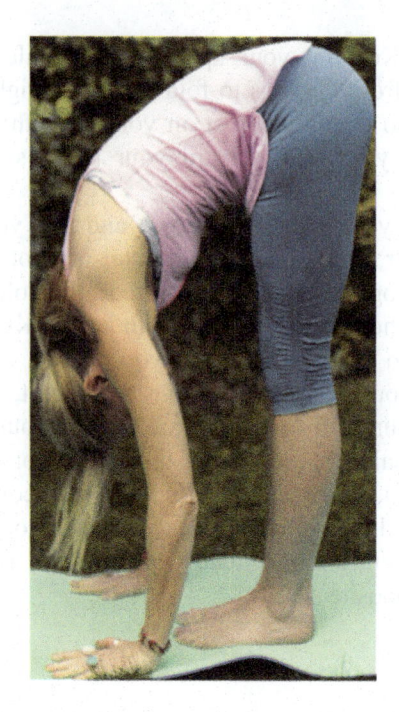

STANDING FORWARD BEND OR UTTANASANA

Forward bends are excellent for calming our nervous system. The posture provides a release of the upper body and soothes the mind through gentle inversion, either when practiced on its own or between postures. This posture stretches your hips, hamstrings and calves, strengthens your thighs and knees, massages your internal organs and helps improve digestion and cleanses mucus from the lungs, relaxes your central nervous system and helps calm your mind, helps relieve stress, headaches, fatigue and insomnia; helps relieve symptoms of menopause and is therapeutic for osteoporosis.

As you stand in Mountain Pose (Tadasana), place your hands on your hips and inhale. As you exhale, soften your knees and fold slowly forward from your hips. Counterbalance your body weight by moving your tailbone

and hips back slightly as the body leans forward. Keep your knees soft so your sit bones point up to the ceiling and your hip points roll forward into the upper thighs.

Rest your hands on the ground beside your feet or hold onto your elbows. Ensure that your feet are still parallel (second and middle toes pointing forward). Hollow out your belly and encourage the chest bone to float down to the top of your feet and increase the space between your pubis and your chest bone. Feel that the fold comes from your hip joint and not from rounding of your lower back.

If the hamstrings feel ease in this stetch, slowly extend your knees more while pushing your sit bones up to the ceiling.

Root into the heels as you slightly turn the top of the thighs inwards. This inwards rotation of your thighs aligns and isolates more of the inner hamstring lines.

Let your head dangle so the crown of your head reaches down to the floor so your gaze is through the legs. Hold for several slow breaths.

To exit, contract your abdominal and core muscles.

As you inhale, place your hands on your hips, soften your knees, and reach your chest far forward. Rise up from your hips keeping your back long. Keep the length between the pubis and chest bone. Continue to lengthen your torso as you come up to standing.

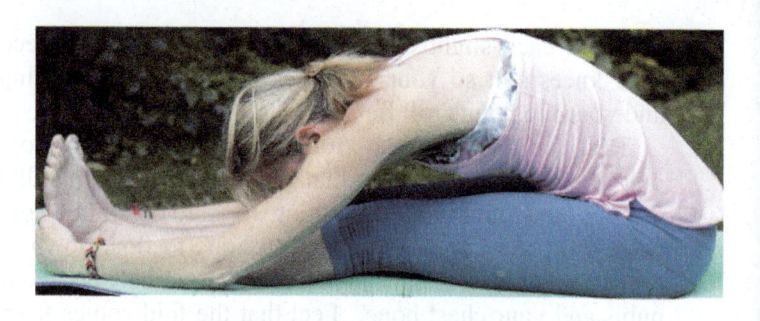

SEATED FORWARD BEND OR PASCHIMOTTANASANA

This asana stretches the hamstring, spine and lower back, calms the mind and relieves stress and anxiety, improves digestion, relieves symptoms of PMS and menopause, reduces fatigue and stimulates the liver, kidneys, ovaries, and uterus. Forward and backbends are great for removing anger, betrayal and all other negative emotions that cause spinal tension. This pose also helps increase awareness by releasing energies that cloud clear thought.

STEP BY STEP

Beginning in the staff pose, raise arms up to the sky, and then bow your upper body down over your upper legs. Our hands rest softly on our legs or feet, wherever they can reach, and little by little the central channel of the spine gives way to the sweet pull of gravity. In forward bends, we invite a calming of the mind – the monkey mind with all of its worries and frets, its many variations of 'what ifs'.

Just for this moment, be completely present. The future lies far away from the next inhalation and exhalation, and it is not yours to fret over or attempt to control. Trust your strong legs, now connected to the ground beneath them, to support you in letting go fully with your upper body. Surrender the worries clouding your sky mind, allow yourself to go deeper into the physical fold, and open up to the vast expanse of peace that has been waiting patiently to bless you.

IMPATIENCE/IRRITABILITY

Are you there yet? Why can't you have it all now? Delaying gratification is what the next generation needs to learn to do. The forty/fifty somethings have been the Generation Fast Food. Have it all now, buying on credit stuff and experience they were unable to afford. Being more considered and pausing before you do anything is another way of saying mindfulness. Being reflective on yourself, holding a mirror up to yourself. I wrote novels which are fictionalised accounts of parts of my life and they are essentially mirrors to my behaviour, thoughts and feelings. If you wrote yourself as a character would you find yourself impatient or irritable?

Observe yourself, don't judge yourself. When you become less impatient, you open up a lot more about yourself and become more considered, more proactive and structured with everything in life from your relationship with yourself, your loved ones and with money and time. Here are some suggested postures. Also see those good for jet lag.

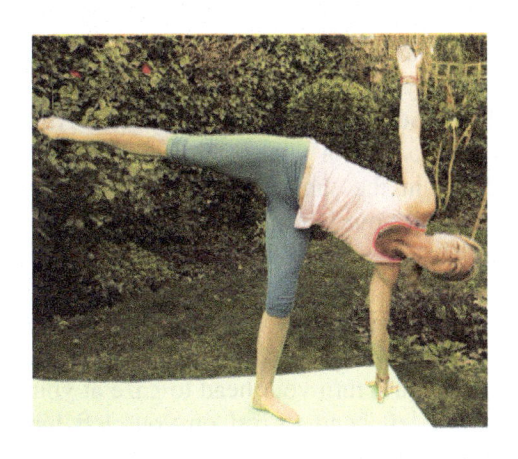

HALF MOON POSE OR ARDHA CHANDRASANA

This asana quiets the mind yet brings awareness. Half Moon is a balancing posture with one leg raised 90 degrees and one hand on the floor or on a block. Balancing poses take our attention from our mind and into our body, expands your chest and shoulders, increases the mobility of your hip joints, increases neck mobility, lengthens your spinal muscles, strengthens and tones the muscles of your thighs and calves, stretches your hamstrings and groin muscles and increases proprioception (the sense of position in space) of the feet and ankles.

STEP BY STEP

Do not practice Half Moon Pose if you have low blood pressure or are currently experiencing headaches, insomnia, or diarrhoea. Those with neck injuries should not turn their heads to face the top hand, but should continue looking straight ahead. Always work within your own range of limits and abilities. If you have any medical concerns, talk with your doctor before practicing yoga.

Begin by standing at the top of your mat. Turn to the left and step your feet wide apart. Extend your arms out to the sides at shoulder-height. Your feet should be as far apart as your wrists. Rotate your right (front) foot 90 degrees, so your front foot's toes point to the top of the mat. Turn your left foot's toes slightly in. Align your front heel with the arch of your back foot. Reach through your right hand in the same direction that your right foot is pointed. Shift your left hip back, and then fold sideways at the hip. Rest your right hand on your outer right shin or ankle. If you are more flexible, place your fingertips on the floor. You can also place your hand on a block. Align your shoulders so your left shoulder is directly above your right shoulder. Gently turn your head to gaze at your left thumb. Bring your left hand to rest on your left hip. Turn your head to look at the floor.

Then, bend your right knee and step your left foot 6-12 inches closer to your right foot. Place your right hand's fingertips on the floor in front of your right foot. Press firmly into your right hand and foot. Straighten your right leg while simultaneously lifting your left leg. Work toward bringing your left leg parallel to the floor, or even higher than your hips. Reach actively through your left heel. Do not lock your right leg's knee. Keep your right foot's toes and kneecap facing in the direction of your head.

Stack your top hip directly over your bottom hip, and open your torso to the left. Then extend your left arm and point your fingertips directly toward the sky. If you can balance comfortably there, turn your head and gaze at your left thumb.

Draw your shoulder blades firmly into your back. Lengthen your tailbone toward your left heel.

Hold for up to one minute. To release, lower your left leg as you exhale. Return to Extended Triangle Pose. Inhale and press firmly through your left heel as you lift your torso. Lower your arms. Turn to the left, reversing the position of your feet, and repeat for the same length of time on the opposite side.

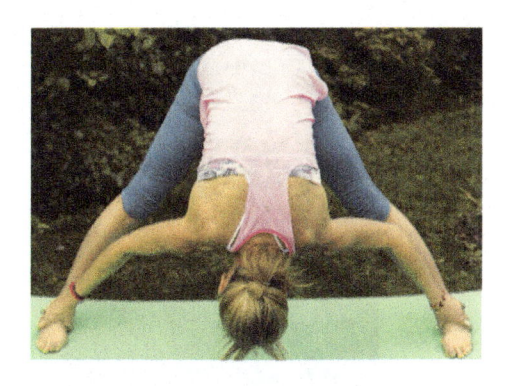

WIDE LEGGED FORWARD BEND OR PRASARITA PADOTTANASANA

This pose is restorative for fatigue, headache, anxiety and mild depression. It also helps to soothe the nervous system because it elongates the spine and re-balances the pressure of the meningeal system around the spinal cord and brain

STEP BY STEP

From star pose, pivot toes slightly inward, firmly press the inside edges of feet down as you lift kneecaps up, firming thighs. Place hands on hip creases. Inhale, lengthen spine and slightly lift chest, and then exhale and fold forward bringing hands to the ground in line with toes. Lift hip bones up and lengthen spine down. Relax neck and jaw, releasing head toward the Earth. Hold for five to eight diaphragmatic breaths.

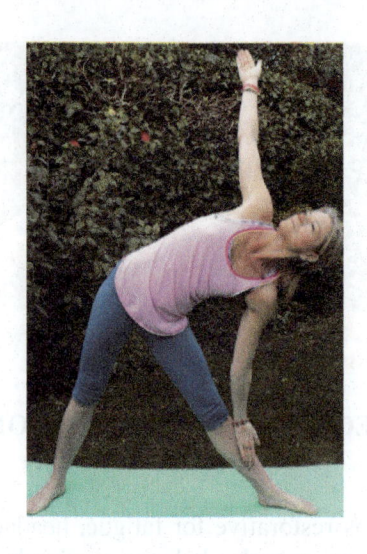

TRIANGLE POSE OR TRIKONASANA

Triangle pose supports digestion and is therapeutic for stress and anxiety. From star pose, pivot your right foot forward to face the front, short end of the mat. While grounding down firmly through the outside edge of your back foot, begin to firm both thighs, lifting kneecaps up. Reach arms to a "T" shape parallel to the floor, gazing over the right middle finger. Inhale and reach right arm forward, lengthening torso over right leg. Exhale and release right hand to the Earth, ankle, shin or yoga block.

Draw the left shoulder down and back while extending left hand up parallel with the right. Right hand stretches down while left hand stretches up, spreading chest, heart and lungs.

Focus on rotating the torso and belly organs toward the sky, twisting from the solar plexus. Keep both thighs engaged and kneecaps lifted.

Hold for five to eight diaphragmatic breaths, and then on an inhalation, press down with right foot and lift up as if the left hand is pulling you up.

STEP BY STEP

From Warrior II, straighten your front leg (the right leg in this case). Reach the right arm towards the front of the room, engaging your right thigh as you go. Drop your right hand down onto your shin or ankle. If you are more open, bring your right hand to the floor on the inside or outside the right foot. Do whichever one feels most comfortable. The left shoulder stacks on top of the right one as you open your chest, reaching the left fingertips towards the ceiling while keeping your left shoulder rooted in its socket.

Take your gaze up toward your left fingertips. Draw the right thigh muscles upwards, deepening the crease in your right hip. Microbend your right knee. Repeat with your left leg forward.

Beginners: bring your right hand higher up on your leg or place a block on the floor under your hand. It is more important to keep your right leg straight than to bring your right hand to the floor. Do not rest your hand directly on your knee, though, as this creates too much pressure on the knee.

RISING ABOVE EGO/VANITY

All balancing postures are excellent for rising above ego. So think Warrior Three (Virabhadrasana Dwi), Eagle Pose (Gorkasana), and side plank. Here are a few more.

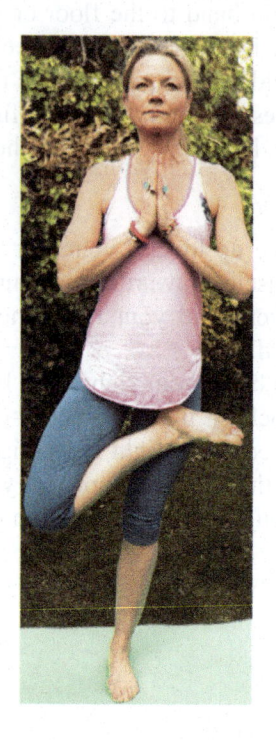

TREE POSE OR VRKSASANA

Improves focus and sense of balance. Supports a feeling of connection with the Earth and current environment. Starting in mountain pose, begin to shift weight onto left foot, bending right knee to bring your right foot and ankle to your calf or inner thigh of left leg. Focus eyes on the ground three to five feet in front of you. If you have a hard time balancing, rest one or both hands against a wall.

Encourage both hips to be in a neutral position, parallel to the floor. Bring palms to touch at your heart's centre, interlacing middle, ring and pinkie fingers, leaving index fingers and thumbs extended. Press left foot firmly into the ground. Inhale and extend arms overhead, lengthening up. Hold for eight to ten diaphragmatic breaths, then on an exhalation return to mountain pose and repeat on opposite side.

STEP BY STEP

Starting in mountain pose begin to shift weight into left foot, bending right knee to bring your right foot and ankle to your calf or inner thigh of left leg.

Focus eyes on the Earth three to five feet in front of you. If you have a hard time balancing, rest one or both hands against a wall. Encourage both hips to be in a neutral position, parallel to floor.

Bring palms to touch at your heart's centre interlacing middle, ring and pinkie fingers leaving index fingers and thumbs extended. Press left foot firmly into the ground.

Inhale and extend arms overhead lengthening up. Hold for eight to 10 diaphragmatic breaths then on an exhale return to mountain pose and repeat on opposite side.

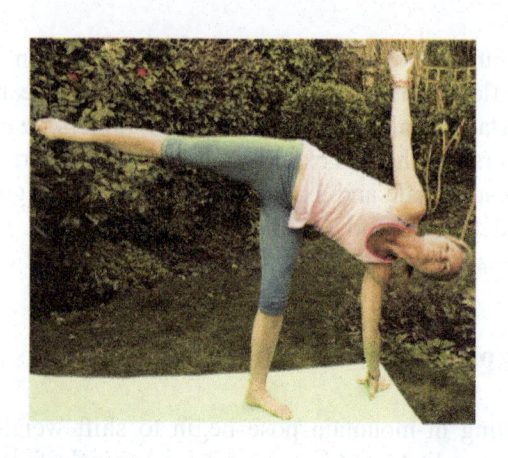

HALF MOON POSE OR ARDHA CHANDRASANA

This asana quiets the mind yet brings awareness. Half Moon is a balancing posture with one leg raised 90 degrees and one hand on the floor or on a block. Balancing poses take our attention from our mind and into our body, expands your chest and shoulders, increases mobility of your hip joints, increases neck mobility, lengthens your spinal muscles, strengthens and tones muscles of your thighs and calves, stretches your hamstrings and groin muscles and increases proprioception (the sense of position in space) of the feet and ankles.

STEP BY STEP

Do not practice Half Moon Pose if you have low blood pressure or are currently experiencing headaches, insomnia, or diarrhoea. Those with neck injuries should not turn their heads to face the top hand, but should continue looking straight ahead. Always work within your own range of limits and abilities. If you have any medical concerns, talk with your doctor before practicing yoga.

Begin by standing at the top of your mat. Turn to the left and step your feet wide apart. Extend your arms out to the sides at shoulder-height. Your feet should be as far apart as your wrists. Rotate your right (front) foot 90 degrees, so your front foot's toes point to the top of the mat. Turn your left foot's toes slightly in. Align your front heel with the arch of your back foot. Reach through your right hand in the same direction that your right foot is pointed. Shift your left hip back, and then fold sideways at the hip. Rest your right hand on your outer right shin or ankle. If you are more flexible, place your fingertips on the floor. You can also place your hand on a block.

Align your shoulders so your left shoulder is directly above your right shoulder. Gently turn your head to gaze at your left thumb.

Bring your left hand to rest on your left hip. Turn your head to look at the floor. Then, bend your right knee and step your left foot 6-12 inches closer to your right foot. Place your right hand's fingertips on the floor in front of your right foot.

Press firmly into your right hand and foot. Straighten your right leg while simultaneously lifting your left leg. Work toward bringing your left leg parallel to the floor, or even higher than your hips.

Reach actively through your left heel. Do not lock your right leg's knee. Keep your right foot's toes and kneecap facing in the direction of your head.

Stack your top hip directly over your bottom hip, and open your torso to the left. Then extend your left arm and point your fingertips directly toward the sky. If you can balance comfortably there, turn your head and gaze at your left thumb.

Draw your shoulder blades firmly into your back. Lengthen your tailbone toward your left heel.

Hold for up to one minute. To release, lower your left leg as you exhale. Return to Extended Triangle Pose.

Inhale and press firmly through your left heel as you lift your torso. Lower your arms. Turn to the left, reversing the position of your feet, and repeat for the same length of time on the opposite side.

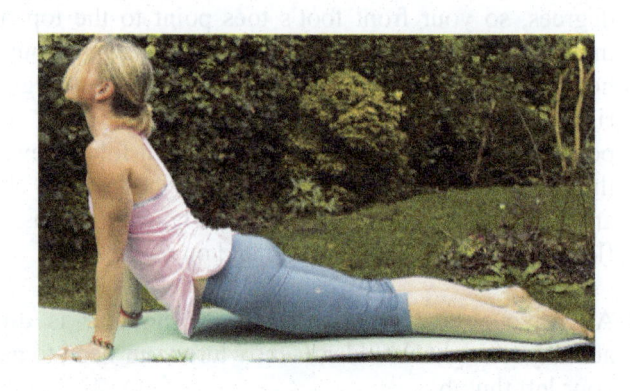

COBRA POSE OR BHUJANGASANA

This posture strengthens your back muscles and arms, increases the flexibility of your spine stretches your chest, shoulders, lungs, and abdomen, and stretches and massages your internal organs and firms your buttocks.

STEP BY STEP

Lie prone on the floor. Stretch your legs back, tops of the feet on the floor. Spread your hands on the floor under your shoulders. Hug the elbows back into your body.

Press the tops of the feet and thighs and the pubis firmly into the floor.

On an inhalation, begin to straighten the arms to lift the chest off the floor, going only to the height at which you can maintain a connection through your pubis to your legs. Press the tailbone toward the pubis and lift the pubis toward the navel. Narrow the hip points. Firm but don't harden the buttocks.

Firm the shoulder blades against the back, puffing the side ribs forward. Lift through the top of the sternum but avoid pushing the front ribs forward, which only hardens the lower back. Distribute the backbend evenly throughout the entire spine.

Hold the pose anywhere from 15 to 30 seconds, breathing easily. Release back to the floor with an exhalation.

VENGEFUL/HATEFUL

Any posture to do with nurturing the heart chakra, the throat chakra and sacrum will help with feelings of revenge. Forward bends and backward bends are particularly good. So think camel posture (Ushtrasana) and seated forward bends (Paschimottanasana). Here are a few more.

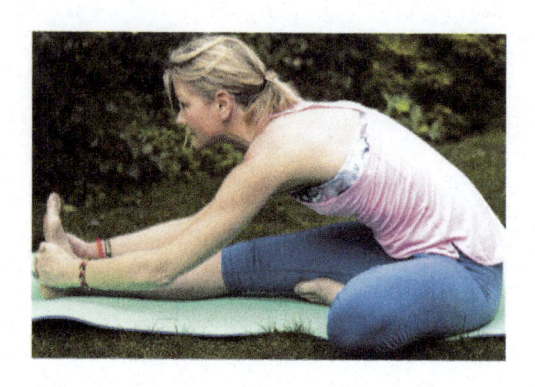

HEAD TO KNEE POSE OR JANU SIRSASANA

This posture stretches your spine, back muscles, hamstrings and groin, massages and stimulates your internal organs like the liver and kidneys, improves digestion and helps heal gastric ailments. It also calms the mind and central nervous system.

STEP BY STEP

Avoid practicing this pose if you are currently suffering from asthma or diarrhoea. Students with back or knee injuries should only practice this pose with the guidance of an experienced and knowledgeable teacher.
Always work within your own range of limits and abilities. If you have any medical concerns, talk with your doctor before practicing yoga.

Sit on the edge of a firm blanket, with your legs extended in front of you in Staff Pose (Dandasana). Bring the sole of your left foot to the inside of your right thigh.

Align the centre of your torso with your right leg (a mild twist). Keeping your spine long, exhale as you hinge forward from the hips to fold over your right leg. Imagine your torso coming to rest on your right thigh, rather than reaching your nose toward your knee (so bend at your waist). Draw your right thigh down and flex your foot. Hold onto your right leg's shin, ankle, or foot. You can also wrap a yoga strap or towel around the sole of your right foot and hold it firmly with both hands.

Keep the front of your torso long; do not round your back. Let your belly touch your thigh first, and then your chest. Your head and nose should touch your leg last.

With each inhalation, lengthen the front torso. With each exhalation, fold deeper.

Hold for 30 seconds. To release the pose, draw your tailbone toward the floor as you inhale and lift your torso.

Extend your left leg. Repeat the pose on the opposite side.

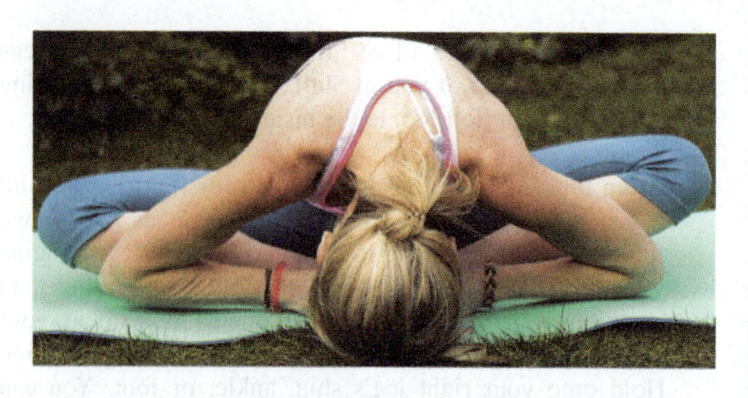

BUTTERFLY POSE/BOUND ANGLE POSE OR BADDHA KONASANA

This asana stretches the inner thighs, groin and knees, stimulates the heart and improves the circulation, stimulates abdominal organs, ovaries, prostate gland and bladder, massages your internal organs and improves digestive circulation, helps reduce menstrual symptoms and discomfort and soothes sciatica pain.

STEP BY STEP

The posture is named Baddha Konasana because of the way it is carried out – both the feet tucked close to the groin, clasped tightly with the hands as though tied or bound together in a particular angle. It is also popularly known as the Butterfly Pose because of the movement of the legs during the posture, giving the appearance of a butterfly flapping its wings. The posture is also sometimes known as the Cobbler Pose as it resembles the sitting position of a cobbler at work. How to do Butterfly Pose (Baddha Konasana): Sit with your spine erect and legs spread straight out. Now bend your knees and bring your feet towards the pelvis. The soles of your feet should touch each other. Grab your feet tightly with your hands. You may place the hands underneath the feet for support. Make an effort to bring the heels as close to the genitals as possible. Take a deep breath in. Breathing out, press the thighs and knees downward towards the floor. Make a gentle effort to keep pressing them downward.

Now start flapping both the legs up and down like the wings of a butterfly. Start slow and gradually increase the speed. Keep breathing normally throughout.

Fly higher and higher, as fast as you comfortably can. Slow down and then stop. Take a deep breath in and as you exhale, bend forward, keeping the chin up and spine erect.

Press your elbows on the thighs or on the knees, pushing the knees and thighs closer to the floor.

Feel the stretch in the inner thighs and take long, deep breaths, relaxing the muscles more and more.

Take a deep breath in and bring the torso up. As you exhale, gently release the posture. Straighten the legs out in front of you and relax.

JETLAG

Jetlag entails anxiety, stress, impatience, irritability and imbalance. These postures help and can also be done (as shown in the photographs) at the airport. Others, I promise you, will join in.

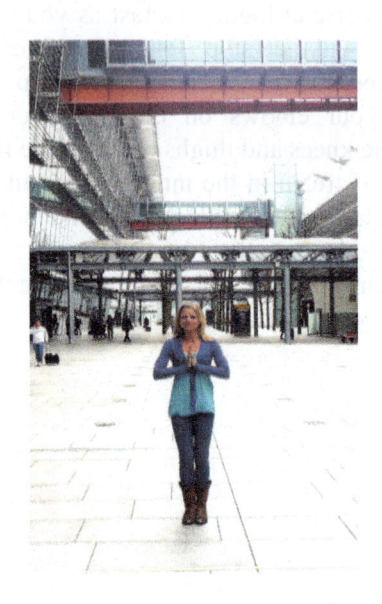

MOUNTAIN POSE OR TADASANA

This is a gentle way to get acquainted with your current atmosphere and improve posture. Stand with feet approximately hip-width distance apart, with spine tall and shoulders relaxed away from ears. Feel your feet on the Earth as you press them firmly into the ground, balancing your weight evenly.

Align centre of skull over centre of pelvis and release arms on either side of torso with palms facing forward.

Relax facial muscles, throat and tongue as you begin to focus on inhaling and exhaling. On the inhalation, breath down into diaphragm and fill to top of lungs.

On exhalation, release breath from top of the lungs to the bottom, releasing your diaphragm last.

This is called diaphragmatic breathing.

Repeat 12 times until you feel grounded and connected to the present moment, taking in the environment around you, feelings, sounds, etc.

STEP BY STEP

This is a gentle way to get acquainted with your current atmosphere and improve posture.

Stand with feet approximately hip-width distance apart, with spine tall and shoulders relaxed away from ears.

Feel your feet on the Earth as you press them firmly into the ground balancing your weight evenly.

Align centre of skull over centre of pelvis and release arms on either side of torso with palms facing forward.

Relax facial muscles, throat and tongue as you begin to focus on inhaling and exhaling.

On the inhale, breath down into diaphragm and fill to top of lungs. On exhale, release breath from top of the lungs to the bottom, releasing your diaphragm last. This is called diaphragmatic breathing.

Repeat 12 times until you feel grounded and connected to the present moment, taking in the environment around you, feelings, sounds, etc.

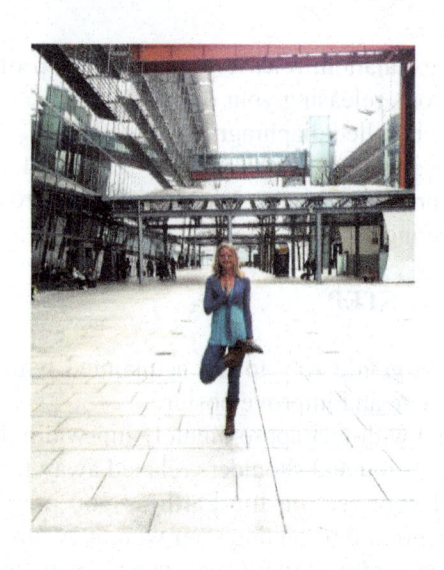

TREE POSE OR VRKSASANA

Improves focus and sense of balance. Supports a feeling of connection with the Earth and current environment. Starting in mountain pose, begin to shift weight into left foot, bending right knee to bring your right foot and ankle to your calf or inner thigh of left leg. Focus eyes on the ground three to five feet in front of you. If you have a hard time balancing, rest one or both hands against a wall. Encourage both hips to be in a neutral position, parallel to floor.

Bring palms to touch at your heart's centre, interlacing middle, ring and pinkie fingers, leaving index fingers and thumbs extended. Press left foot firmly into the ground. Inhale and extend arms overhead, lengthening up. Hold for eight to ten diaphragmatic breaths (see mountain pose), then on an exhalation return to mountain pose and repeat on opposite side.

STEP BY STEP

Starting in mountain pose (above) begin to shift weight into left foot bending right knee to bring your right foot and ankle to your calf or inner thigh of left leg.

Focus eyes on the Earth three to five feet in front of you. If you have a hard time balancing, rest one or both hands against a wall. Encourage both hips to be in a neutral position, parallel to floor.

Bring palms to touch at your heart's centre interlacing middle, ring and pinkie fingers leaving index fingers and thumbs extended. Press left foot firmly into the ground.

Inhale and extend arms overhead lengthening up. Hold for eight to 10 diaphragmatic breaths (see mountain pose), then on an exhalation return to mountain pose and repeat on opposite side.

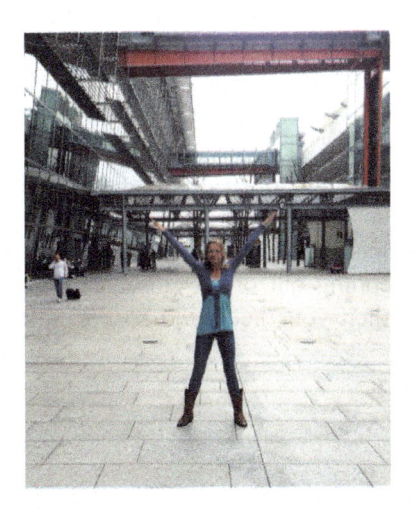

STAR POSE FOR JET LAG YOGA

From a standing position, step feet out about three-and-a-half to four feet apart, coming into a wide-leg stance with feet parallel. Firmly press both feet down as you lift kneecaps up, firming thighs. Inhale, reach arms overhead, and then exhale releasing arms to a "T" shape parallel to the ground. Draw bellybutton up and back toward spine, activating your core and helping to keep bottom rib cage from bowing forward. Hold for eight to ten diaphragmatic breaths, and then release arms and heel-toe feet together coming back into a comfortable standing position.

STEP BY STEP

This pose encourages a sense of adaptability to new locations and energises the body.

From a standing position, step feet out about three-and-a-half to four feet apart, coming into a wide-leg stance with feet parallel.

Firmly press both feet down as you lift kneecaps up, firming thighs.

Inhale, reach arms overhead, and then exhale releasing arms to a "T" shape parallel to the Earth.

Draw bellybutton up and back toward spine activating your core and helping to keep bottom rib cage from bowing forward.

Hold for eight to 10 diaphragmatic breaths, and then release arms and heel-toe feet together, coming back into a comfortable standing position. (Heel-toe means instead of harshly stepping out of the pose, inch your heel in, then your toe, then your heel, and so on until your feet meet again.)

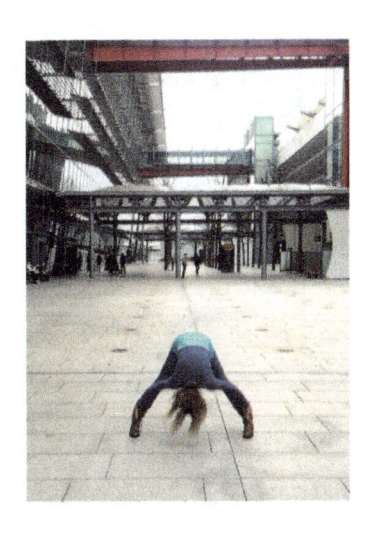

WIDE LEGGED FORWARD BEND FOR JET LAG

This pose is restorative for fatigue, headache, anxiety and mild depression. It also helps to soothe the nervous system because it elongates the spine and re-balances the pressure of the meningeal system around the spinal cord and brain.

From star pose, pivot toes slightly inward, firmly press the inside edges of feet down as you lift kneecaps up firming thighs.

Place hands on hip creases. Inhale, lengthen spine and slightly lift chest, and then exhale and fold forward bringing hands to the ground in line with toes. Lift hip bones up and lengthen spine down. Relax neck and jaw, releasing head toward the Earth. Hold for five to eight diaphragmatic breaths.

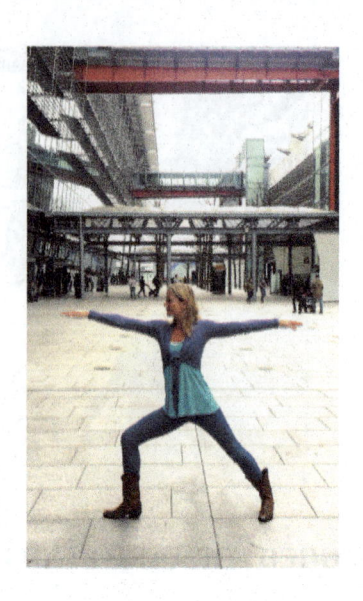

WARRIOR II FOR JET LAG

A powerful stretch for the legs, groins, and chest, Warrior II also increases stamina. It helps to relieve backaches, and stimulates healthy digestion.

This is a deep hip-opening pose that strengthens the muscles in the thighs and buttocks. It tones the abdomen, ankles, and arches of the feet. This pose also opens the chest and shoulders, improving breathing capacity and increasing circulation throughout the body. It is also known to be therapeutic for flat feet, sciatica, infertility, and osteoporosis.

More than just a physical posture, Warrior II increases your ability to concentrate. As you hone your gaze, you direct your mind clearly and with intention. Distractions disappear and your energy becomes powerful and focused.

Do not practice Warrior II if you have a recent hip, knee, or shoulder injury, or if you are experiencing diarrhoea or high blood pressure. Those with neck injuries should not turn their head to face the front hand (in step 10). Always work within your own range of limits and abilities. If you have any medical concerns, talk with your doctor before practicing yoga.

STEP BY STEP

Stand in Tadasana. With an exhalation, step or lightly jump your feet 3 1/2 to 4 feet apart. Raise your arms parallel to the floor and reach them actively out to the sides, shoulder blades wide, palms down.

Turn your right foot slightly to the right and your left foot out to the left 90 degrees. Align the left heel with the right heel. Firm your thighs and turn your left thigh outward so that the centre of the left knee cap is in line with the centre of the left ankle.

Exhale and bend your left knee over the left ankle, so that the shin is perpendicular to the floor. If possible, bring the left thigh parallel to the floor. Anchor this movement of the left knee by strengthening the right leg and pressing the outer right heel firmly to the floor.

Stretch the arms away from the space between the shoulder blades, parallel to the floor. Don't lean the torso over the left thigh: Keep the sides of the torso equally long and the shoulders directly over the pelvis. Press the tailbone slightly toward the pubis. Turn the head to the left and look out over the fingers.

Stay for 30 seconds to a minute. Inhale to come up. Reverse the feet and repeat for the same length of time to the left.

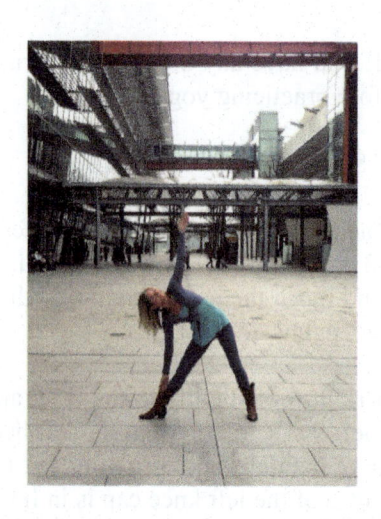

TRIANGLE POSE FOR JET LAG

Triangle pose supports digestion and is therapeutic for stress and anxiety. From star pose, pivot your right foot forward to face the front, short end of the mat. While grounding down firmly through the outside edge of your back foot, begin to firm both thighs, lifting kneecaps up.

Reach arms to a "T" shape parallel to the floor, gazing over the right middle finger. Inhale and reach right arm forward, lengthening torso over right leg.

Exhale and release right hand to the Earth, ankle, shin or yoga block. Draw the left shoulder down and back while extending left hand up parallel with the right. Right hand stretches down while left hand stretches up, spreading chest, heart and lungs.

Focus on rotating the torso and belly organs toward the sky, twisting from the solar plexus. Keep both thighs engaged and kneecaps lifted. Hold for five to eight diaphragmatic breaths, and then on an inhale, press down with right foot and lift up as if the left hand is pulling you up.

STEP BY STEP

From Warrior II, straighten your front leg (the right leg in this case).

Reach the right arm towards the front of the room, engaging your right thigh as you go.

Drop your right hand down onto your shin or ankle. If you are more open, bring your right hand to the floor on the inside or outside the right foot. Do whichever one feels most comfortable.

The left shoulder stacks on top of the right one as you open your chest, reaching the left fingertips towards the ceiling while keeping your left shoulder rooted in its socket.

Take your gaze up toward your left fingertips.

Draw the right thigh muscles upwards, deepening the crease in your right hip.

Microbend your right knee. Repeat with your left leg forward.

Beginners: Bring your right hand higher up on your leg or place a block on the floor under your hand. It is more important to keep your right leg straight than to bring your right hand to the floor. Do not rest your hand directly on your knee, though, as this creates too much pressure on the knee.

CHAPTER FOUR

THE YOGA A TO Z

A

Age
Yoga is something anyone may practice. From five to ninety five year old. There's a surge in parents now encouraging children to practice yoga which is excellent both for their bodies as well as their spirit and mind. It needs to be fun and diverting. For the middle aged, it's more about clearing the mind, and for the elderly, improving the quality of breath.

Astrology
Character traits will impact on how you choose to practice yoga, but regardless of whether you are an air sign (creative/busy mind), or earth sign (grounded but stubborn), fire sign (driven but issues with temper), or water sign (empathetic and emotional), you will benefit from the balancing effect of yoga in as much as you will incorporate all the benefits of the elements – water, fire, earth and air. You need them all and the chakras align themselves with the same elements.

Asanas
The sanskrit for posture.

Ajna Chakra - third eye chakra
Located between the eyebrows at what is known as the third eye. The Ajna means to perceive and command. Its colour is indigo blue. It has two lotus petals here. Its element is light. Its mantra is Sham. Its function is to vitalise the lower brain, the cerebellum, the central nervous system and vision, as well as to perceive patterns and establish one's personal identity.

The body parts it relates to are the cerebellum, left eye, nose, ears and pituitary gland.

Balanced characteristics include being intuitive, perceptive, imaginative, having a good memory, able to visualise, good dream recollection, able to think symbolically.

Negative characteristics include lack of concentration, insensitivity, lack of imagination, poor dream recollection, denial of what is going on around you.

Physically this may emerge in headaches, tension, vision issues.

Healing practices include meditation, guided visualisations, creating visual art, memory skills enhancement, dream work and hypnosis.

Yoga postures which are good for this chakra include PASCHIMOTTANASANA (forward fold), ADHO MUKHA SVANASANA, BALASANA (child's pose), PRASARITA PADOTTANASANA (standing legs wide forward fold), SUPTA BADDHA KONASANA (reclining bound ankle pose), SETU BANDHA SARVANGASANA (supported bridge pose), SAVASANA (corpse pose).

Affirmations relevant to this chakra: I see with love and joy. I see all things clearly. I am open to the wisdom within. I can manifest my vision. I now create a life I love to look at.

Anahata Chakra - heart chakra

Finding the balance in love. Located at the chest, heart and cardiac plexus. The word 'Anahata' means 'unstuck'. Its colour is green. Twelve lotus petals reside here. Its element is air. Its mantra is Yam. Its function is to anchor the life force with the higher self. Energizes blood and physical body with life force or prana and circulates it throughout the body. Its purpose is love and balance.

Body parts it relates to are heart, thymus gland, circulatory system, arms, hands and lungs.

Balanced characteristics include being compassionate, loving, empathetic, self-loving, altruistic, peaceful, balanced and having a good immune system.

Possible negative characteristics include co-dependency, poor boundaries, being demanding, clinging and jealous, repression of love, fear of intimacy, lack of empathy, narcissism, and emotional instability.

Physical malfunctions include disorders of the heart, lungs, thymus, breasts and arms. Shortness of breath, sunken chest, circulation problems, asthma, immune system deficiency, tension between shoulder blades, pain in the chest.

Healing practices include breathing exercises (PRANAYAMA), strengthening of arms, reaching out to others, journaling, self-discovery regarding forgiveness, self-acceptance, emotional release of grief.

Yoga postures to try include NATARAJASANA (dancer pose), ADHO MUKHA SVANASANA (downward facing dog or half dog up wall), PASCHIMOTTANASANA (seated forward fold) UTTANASANA (standing forward fold), BHUJANGASANA (cobra pose) PASASANA (noose pose), GOMUKHASANA (cow face pose), VIRASANA (hero pose), USHTRASANA (camel pose), SETU BANDHA SARVANGASANA (bridge pose), BALASANA (child's pose) SVANASANA (corpse pose).

Affirmations for this chakra are:

I am worthy of love. There is an infinite supply of love. I live in balance with others, joy, joy, joy. I lovingly allow joy to flow through my mind and body and experience.

B

Beauty

Prettiness is in the eye of the beholder. Beauty is transparent to everyone. Before going on a botox fix or trying to change the shape you are and how you look through cosmetic surgery, check out Antonia Mariconda. She is a leading health and beauty journalist offering no nonsense advice to those feeling they are not enough and surgery will somehow fix that. When I was researching for health and anti ageing products and services, she was my guide through the maze of creams, potions, lotions, and procedures. Check out www.thecosmeticcoach.com.

Body dysmorphic disorder
BDD is relatively common – it affects about one in 100 people (significantly more than schizophrenia; slightly more than anorexia). It typically starts in early teens and affects boys as frequently as girls. The causes of BDD are still unknown. 'We know it runs in families' and that there is a strong genetic component, but that doesn't explain the whole picture,' Dr Mataix-Cols says, listing such factors as 'appearance-related teasing' and bullying. 'It's not clear if they simply trigger a pre-existing vulnerability or whether they have a proper causal effect.'

Yoga is effective in overcoming self-esteem issues which relate to body issues. There is no judgement or competition – although ironically there are 'yoga competitions', but yoga in class or in personal training has no competition – especially with self. Yoga is about finding balance, in mind, body, spirit and emotion and learning self compassion. **For more information about BDD www.ifeelugly.info**

Best
As in being the best. Doing your best. Don't even think about 'best'. There is no concept of best. There is no judgement with yoga, no competition with others or with self.

Balance
What yoga is all about – emotional, spiritual, physical balance. Balancing postures are good for improving

memory, rising above ego (i.e. getting over yourself if you have high self esteem issues) and concentration.

C

Chakras
The chakras are essentially a deeper model for understanding ourselves, a way to expand our notion of reality. 'Chakra' means 'Wheel' or a spinning vortex of energy that is beyond the external physical body, like 'doorways' to our sense of ourselves and our sense of reality in our psyche. The Chakras are where we assimilate, receive and distribute our life energy. When we begin an inward focus towards our true selves, and begin to make effective changes within ourselves, instead of focusing on our negativity, we ascend towards our hearts being full of a blissful, compassionate, joyful experience of every moment in our life.

Within the theory of the Chakras, we look towards Tantra, which explores the essential unity of reality – the creation of the universe through the dynamic interplay of two powerful forces: Shiva and Shakti. These represent duality: light/dark, soft/loud, male/female. The Tantric path is to realise through experience that the world of duality is only an illusion and that everything is divine and connected.

There are seven Chakras, located through the centre of the spine in Sushumna Nadi, the main energy channel in the body, meaning 'ray of light'. When Sushumna Nadi is purified through the Chakras, Shakti energy moves up the spine to re-unite with the source of all creativity, Shiva.

The lower three Chakras relate to your self-image and the external world. At the heart centre we being to focus inside, and the upper three Chakras relate to rising above the ego towards our spiritual self.

Most of us live within the lower three chakras – the basics. This is where we consider what we will eat and when, where our home is, who our partner is and how we feel secure, then our sense of sensuality, creativity and how we feel fulfilled in our lives; we then move on to our ego-identity and sense of self; how we are perceived by others, our self-esteem.

Living a more yogic life, we move beyond these basic thoughts and into the place of our spiritual body in asana and pranayama practice; we can then begin to align these subtle energies to heal ourselves, to move beyond the mundane everyday existence of food, money, power towards our true nature.

The whole idea behind the asana practice is that these subtle energies move towards subhuman Nadi, where the Chakras are located, and prana is then powerful, spirited and aligned. When the body is aligned correctly with prana, the healing qualities can take place and one can feel better. It is this 'feeling' that is key to yoga; many westerners are shut off from their feelings, often blotting out true feelings with droning, drugs, repetitive negative behaviour, unfulfilling relationships, anger, blame. The whole purpose of yoga is to subtly shift the energy away from these choices towards choices that are healing, positive, enlightened, sattvic.

Each Chakra has a related Bija Mantra, or seed sound – these are powerful tools for self healing. To chant/sing the Bija Mantra is to purify that Chakra and move up to the next. Also, when we sing we create vibration not eh roof of the mouth, where we have 84 meridian points. The Bija Mantras are in nature uplifting and healing.

LAM	Mulhadara Chakra	Base of the spine
VAM	Svadhisthanda Chakra	Sacrum

RAM	Manipura Chakra	Navel and solar plexus
YAM	Anahata Chakra	Heart centre
HAM	Vishuddha Chakra	Throat centre
OM	Ajna Chakra	Centre of the eyebrows
OM (silent)	Sahasrara Chakra	Crown of the head

The 'thousand petal lotus' is the Sahasrara Chakra, which relates to the Pineal and Pituitary Glands. The latter is called the 'Master Gland' because it is capable of recharging the entire body and mind on all levels. The pineal gland is the seat of memory, therefore a blessing as it can recall past mistakes, but also a curse as the same mistakes are then made over again until the balance is attained.

Competition
Yoga is not competitive. Those who make it competitive are not doing yoga. They are doing exercise with stretching.

Child's pose
This looks a very restful pose, but it elongates the spine and allows you to listen to your breath. This posture, as well as cow and cat pose, is effective when you wish to halt the practice. Don't just stop, go into child pose. You will continue your meditation even if you stop your movement.

Colour
What to wear? Think of colour and wear it – it will help you to visualise it. Turquoise is good for calming, protection and healing. Warm red for energy. Steer clear of blue reds and silver. Each chakra has a colour so work with those colours (crown chakra, purple; throat chakra, blue; third eye chakra, indigo; heart chakra, green; sacrum

chakra, orange; solar plexus and navel chakra, yellow; base chakra red). Try to pick those colours to wear but keep clothes loose fitting.   Colours also have meaning.

RED:
warmth, love, anger, danger, boldness, excitement, speed, strength, energy, determination, desire, passion, courage, socialism

PINK:
feminine, love, caring, nurture

ORANGE:
cheerfulness, low cost, affordability, enthusiasm, stimulation, creativity, aggression, food, halloween, liberal (politics)

YELLOW:
attention-grabbing, comfort, liveliness, cowardice, hunger, optimism, overwhelm, Summer, comfort, liveliness, intellect, happiness, energy, conflict

GREEN:
durability, reliability, environmental, luxurious, optimism, well-being, nature, calm, relaxation, Spring, safety, honesty, optimism, harmony, freshness

BLUE:
peace, professionalism, loyalty, reliability, honor, trust, melancholia, boredom, coldness, Winter, depth, stability, professionalism, conservatism

PURPLE:
power, royalty, nobility, elegance, sophistication, artificial, luxury, mystery, royalty, elegance, magic

GREY:
conservatism, traditionalism, intelligence, serious, dull, uninteresting

BROWN:
relaxing, confident, casual, reassuring, nature, earthy, solid, reliable, genuine, Autumn, endurance

BLACK:
Elegance, sophistication, formality, power, strength, illegality, depression, morbidity, night, death

WHITE:
Cleanliness, purity, newness, virginity, peace, innocence, simplicity, sterility, snow, ice, cold

Calm
Do you know how to be calm? What does calm mean to you? Think of the things in life that make you calm. Not 'things' as in objects, but spaces, places, people, smells, tastes. The sensual world. Think of these things and focus on these positive images. And then focus on your breath, every night before you go to sleep. And don't watch the news. Too negative, focusing on the negative even when there is a positive story to tell. Too depressing – the antithesis of calm.

Choice
Yoga helps you to make decisions. Indecisiveness causes stress and fuddles the brain. Yoga clears the mind, improves decisiveness and eases stress.

D

Dharmas
Sanskrit for the laws of nature, considered both collectively and individually. If the teacher mentions these it will be in relation to how the body, mind and spirit are interlinked as one.

Downward dog
Excellent posture. Good for alleviating anxiety, stress, improving focus and concentration, elongating the spine and hamstrings. This posture works all chakras. Keep the hips high, pushing back with the hands, relaxing the shoulders, lifting up through the hips, lengthening and strengthening the hamstrings and spine. The more you practice, the closer the heels will come to the floor as the hamstrings loosen, and the more relaxed the shoulders, the straighter the spine will become. Place hands so the space

between the fore finger and thumb is facing the front of the mat and elbows are pointing in to one another. This will open up the chest. Keep breath long, strong and even.

Dance
Any form of dance is wonderful for the heart and throat chakras. However, dancers tend to over extend their bodies. The more you practice yoga the more aware you will become of how, when you dance, you open up your heart and throat chakras, but over extend and stretch ligaments which may cause issues when you are older. However, dance is an incredibly joyful form of exercise, use with knowledge of your anatomy and how yoga works the esoteric (emotional) system and you will realise how important dancing in your life is to your sense of wellbeing and joy.

E

Eagle

This is a visualisation which works when you lack energy, confidence, direction and courage. It empowers. Lie on your back in savasana. Close your eyes. If you can place a roller underneath your back (long polystyrene tubes you find in gyms) along your spine to open your chest, that would be great. No worries if you can't. Push your shoulders back into the mat. Breath deeply and slowly.

Visualise yourself as an eagle. Spread your arms out. You are flying over hills and forests. The sky is blue, with a few clouds. Only a few, and the wind is light and pushing you forwards. You look down, and there are villages and towns below you with people rushing around. They look like ants and there are thousands of them, all rushing about, meeting deadlines. You are rising above them. Spread your winds and breath in deeply.

The wind is pushing against you now and its starting to rain. Feel the rain on your wings, in your feathers. Breath in and cut through the wind. Don't turn back. Fly through it. This makes you stronger. You enjoy feeling the rain and wind on your wings. Slice through the wind and the rain and fly higher. Reach higher into the sky. Breath in, and out. Slow and strong. Stretch your wings out (and your arms).

Fly high, up, up into the mountains. Fly around the mountains where the air is thin, but fresh and cool and breath deeper now. Land on top of a mountain, or near the top and gaze around you. You are above the clouds and see through the holes in the clouds the land beneath you. Look to your horizon and see how far you see. The perspective, the enormity of what you have achieved. Breath in that feeling. Be strong, like an eagle. Be brave. Observe like an eagle, don't judge. Rise above the rush of the villages and towns, like the eagle. Be proactive like the eagle. Eagles are predators, they are active not reactive. They are observers.

Observe yourself and breath in this feeling of courage, strength, rising above it and being able to see clearly from the best perspective.

This visualisation is particularly good for those lacking in courage, self confidence and fatigue.

Esoteric
The word esoteric has its roots in the Greek 'esoterikos', a compound of 'within'. This form of anatomy is the subtle anatomy of the body, the knowledge of which is in the ancient Indian yogic texts. Discussing the Chakras and other theories of esoteric anatomy, we use the word 'energy'. In Sanskrit, all existence is a constantly vibrating primordial force field called MAHASHAKTI (meaning Mother Power). The concept of Maha Shakti most accurately describes what we call energy. 'Energy' is

useful to describe the subtle interaction of the vibrating forces at play within each of us, human and animal, which are the very primordial Maha Shakti.

Exhale

Get rid of unwanted energy, stuff you don't need, emotional baggage that is of no use to you. Just get rid of it. Don't take on other people's stuff either.

Ego

Rise above it. It gets in the way with yoga. Do not set out to achieve a goal, rather go with an open mind, you will achieve more. I occasionally ask my students to do as much of the class as they are able with their eyes closed. Not all, but most. They all, without exception, improve posture and alignment and their breath slows and deepens. This is because they do not judge themselves or each other, or feel judged. They just literally 'feel' their way from one posture to another and feel what is right. Which is.

F

Flow

Go with it. Do not think about what you are 'doing' but focus on how the asanas make you feel. Observe the images that come into your mind as you practice. The asanas stimulate the 'truth' within you – i.e those things which you are holding onto which are creating blocks in your system, either in terms of emotional or mental worries or physical ailments. Make note of them and talk to the teacher afterwards about them. They will tell you a lot about yourself.

Food

Don't eat just before yoga but don't starve yourself. Juicing and detoxing are often talked about in the same breath as yoga, but keeping it light is always good.

Breakfast like a king, lunch like a prince, dine like a pauper. That's a good way to eat.

Flexibility
All yoga postures improve flexibility and flexibility improves your sense of wellbeing.

G

Guru
Gurus. This is an interesting one. There will be teachers you will meet who will inspire you but they are teachers. They are there to pass on practice. That is it. They inspire you and inform you. They are not Gods.

Gender
It is a much held belief that women are more flexible than men. However, look at men in some yoga classes and you will realise this is not the case, and with patience men are able to be just as flexible as women. It takes diligence and discipline. In yoga there is no battle of the sexes. There is balance of the sexes, yin and yang. Men will get as much out of yoga as women. I admit when I teach men, I don't mention chakras, dharmas or anything vaguely rainbows and unicorns. They switch off. I focus on the basics of where the pain in their back is and why it may have occurred. Then they usually think I'm a witch.

H

Hippy
Yoga is not the preserve of the Ibiza hippy movement, nor is it exclusive to California, the Himalayas, or India. It is universal. Yes, there are some places more conducive than others. I have taught in a health club where they were playing squash next door and the wall behind me was the wall they bashed the ball against. Not only that, but the language they were using was ripe. Added to which the

acoustics were lousy for music. But it was a wonderful way of testing focus and concentration, although I wouldn't recommend it for every practice.

Height
If you are short, yoga is less challenging than for those who are tall (over five foot eight). Especially if you have short legs or arms, as it means when you are doing head or handstands you have less 'bend'. It sounds silly but it's true. You get a lot of short people practicing yoga because it is allegedly supposed to make you taller (extending the spine and hamstrings). I believe it improves the posture to create the illusion of looking taller, but you are literally walking taller so that is good enough.

Heat
You will generate a lot of heat in the body during yoga. Even learning to breath properly will create heat in the body. Whether its power yoga, Bikram (where you will sweat in 90 degree heat) or Vinyasa, or even the more regimented Hatha and Ashtanga, the asanas are focusing on improving circulation, which in turn warms the body.

Hypnotherapy
This works well with the practice of yoga on emotional issues. I recommend Ailsa Frank.
www.hypnobalance.co.uk or www.ailsafrank.com.
01276683123. She uses effective techniques on a range of emotional issues and specialises in forms of addiction (alcohol, smoking). Also excellent for self esteem issues.

I

Inhale
At the start of each session I usually ask the group to sit cross legged, palms up on the knees, shoulders back, eyes closed. I then ask them to put their left hand on their abdominals and tell them this is where they should be

breathing from. Not the neck. I then ask them to inhale. The inhalation is initially usually light, quite tight and short. When we are in protective mode (which we are most of the time) we breath light and tight. I then ask them to inhale as much as they can, and hold. Then to sniff (inhale again) and hold. Then sniff again and hold. What this is about is when you feel you have filled your legs - you haven't. If you had, you wouldn't be able to fill your lungs any more. I then ask them to exhale for four, then six, then eight seconds each time after they have inhaled. This is easy to practice at home.

Visualising while you inhale. Inhale all the good in. Visualise inhaling all the good in and opening yourself up to it. Just sit down cross legged, palms facing up and open the fingers, opening up to the good around you. Imagine your face opening up like a flower and welcoming in the good like sunshine on your face. Breath in through the nose, from your abdominals and smile. Now doesn't that feel good?

India
Go once to a retreat in India and experience yoga with a guru recommended to you. Take what you want from it, but don't isolate the experience and think nothing else compares. Everyone offers something different. Every culture offers something different. India has a culture that is accepting of death, life pain and balance. That is why it is conducive to the practice of yoga. It is the culture and colour of India rather than the need for joss sticks and excessive heat. Remember that. Remember why it is special. It is not for the reasons you may initially think. And your expectations will be high. After all you have paid all that money to get there.

J

Joss sticks
In practice a good idea, but they make the studio or room you are practicing in very 'heady'. A clear space and naturally sweet smelling is always best to avoid distraction from focusing on your breath. Plus, if you need scent, I use aromatherapy oils at the end of the practice to help focus or enhance the experience.

Judgement
Do not judge yourself or judge others. Do not compare yourself or your practice to the practice of others in the class. It is not a competition.

K

Kisses
There are postures in yoga where you place head to knee or ankle. Rather than just resting the head, kiss the knee or ankle. It's a small gesture of thanks but it works for how grateful we should be to our bodies. They are amazing.

L

Love and light
A lot of spiritual people sign off with this. As in letters or notes or emails. I initially thought it was hippy-speak, but it sums up the elements of inner peace. The ability to know you are loved and are capable of love, and love yourself, and the focus on the light, which embodies positive energy running through and around you however you want to see it – as an energy or as your spirit.

Learning
You never stop learning. It is a continual process. Yoga teachers are continually going to other classes and topping

up their practice. Yoga is an emotional, spiritual and physical journey which are interlinked. The lesson learnt through yoga is there is always more to learn. No one knows it all.

Life experience
The more you have the more you will get from the practice of yoga. Yoga is about clearing the mind and releasing the emotions and realising they are not your 'enemies' as they often treated, but a natural release. When they are released, then the mind is able to function more logically. Compassion for yourself and your vulnerabilities is where it starts, having a sense of identity and self-esteem where it continues, being happy with yourself is where it ends.

M

Manipura Chakra
Located at the navel centre, its colour is yellow. 'Manipura' means 'lustrous gem'. Its element is fire. There are ten lotus petals here. Its gem is amber, topaz or tiger eye. Its Mantra is Ram. Its function is the sympathetic nervous system, digestive processes, and metabolism. It is the place where ego resides. The body parts it relates to are the pancreas, the adrenals, stomach, liver, gall bladder, nervous system and muscles.

If you are balanced in this area, you are responsible, reliable, balanced, warm in personality, confident, appropriately self-disciplined, able to meet challenges, you have a strong sense of your personal power, playfulness and a sense of humour.

If you are out of balance, you take on more than you can handle, you are power hungry. Also issues with anger, fear, hate, competitive, a need to be right, poor self-discipline, low self-esteem and emotionally cold.

Physically this will come out in eating disorders, digestive problems, ulcers, hypoglycaemia, diabetes, muscle spasms, muscular disorders, chronic fatigue, hypertension, disorders of the stomach, pancreas, gall bladder and liver.

Healing practices include stress control, deep relaxation, vigorous exercise, martial arts, pilates, psychotherapy that builds confidence, releases anger, works on shame issues, and strengthens will, encouragement of autonomy.

Yoga poses to work on include BHARADVAJASANA (twist), UTTANASANA (standing forward fold), ADHO MUKHA VIRASANA (Child's Pose) MARICHYASANA (seated forward fold), JATHARA PARIVARTANASANA (revolved abdomen or bent knee twist), SURYA NAMASKAR (sun salutations or modified sun salutations), URDHVA PRASARITA PADASANA (30 60 90 leg lifts) PRANAYAMA (forced exhalation of stale air).

Affirmations for this chakra:

I am at peace. I am calm. I love and approve of myself. This moment is filled with joy. I now choose to experience the sweetness of today. I honour the power within me. The fire within me burns through all blocks and fears. I accomplish tasks easily and effortlessly.

Meditation
This is what yoga is all about. The practice improves our ability to meditate, although yoga is a meditation with movement. Yoga nurtures the ability to stay in one spot, clear mind, calm spirit, right action and be at peace with yourself and the world. Sounds simple but it isn't. If it was, we would all be doing it, but our minds are so busy, so distracted, so on alert, we forget how to be at peace. For excellent practice contact Julie Smith who organises excellent classes in the UK.

Julie Smith
Certified Meditation Expert
Nature Meditations
Website: www.julie-smith.net

Facebook:
http://www.facebook.com/NatureMeditations
Email: julie@julie-smith.net
Phone: +44 (0)7823335833

Mischief
There is so much natural humour in yoga. The asanas have such lyrical names – dolphin pose, cow face pose, hero pose, eagle pose, and there is a playful nature as well (happy baby pose, for example). You do not have to be po faced to do the posture. Not saying you should grin from ear to ear all the way through but don't forget the sense of joy. If Lord Yehudi Menuhin can achieve it, so can you.

Music
Music adds rhythm to the class. It also helps to calm the spirit. If the music is well chosen. If the music has lyrics, no matter how relaxing and chilled, it engages the mind and you focus on the words, not your breath. Music needs to be carefully chosen so it enhances not distracts from the flow.

Mula Bandha
In Sanskrit 'mula' means root, and 'bandha' means 'lock'. To find it, sit, stand, or even be in an asana, and if you are a man contract the area between the anus and the testes. If you are a woman, contract the muscles at the bottom of the pelvic floor behind the cervix. Initially the anal sphincter will also contract, but with time and practice you will be able to hone in on the Mula Bandha region and leave the rest aside. Mula Bandha should be held throughout your entire yoga practice. There are countless reasons, but quite simply think of it as the lock that allows your energy to flow up, not down and out. If your energy is forced to flow up, and stay inside you, for that matter, it will grow exponentially, leaving you with that amazing feeling of 'floating' as you walk out of class. It will also allow you to

float in class, as an engaged Mula Bandha allows you to be lighter on your limbs, and thus lighter on your mat. The lightness prevents you from becoming fatigued when that teacher (me) makes you hold something for what seems like forever and a day or do the umpteenth Chataranga. In a more psychological sense, Mula Bandha stimulates the pelvic nerves, the genital system, the endocrine system and the excretory system. It has also been shown to relieve constipation and depression.

Mirrors
Dancers are always looking at themselves in mirrors to check on alignment and so it should be with yoga, but there is an element of ego involved and also comparing your movement and body to someone else in the room. This detracts focus and hinders balance and breath, so destroys the object of the practice. That's why I ask the class to frequently close their eyes (within reason – I don't want them hurting themselves), but as soon as this happens they breath and balance more effectively. There is no judgement. Use the mirrors to look at the symmetry, not judge how 'good' the movement is. Keep the ego out of it.

N

Neck
Use it, lengthen it, expose it. The English culture is one of keeping the head down; even the phrase 'keep the head down' denotes keeping out of trouble, working hard and with diligence. But it is defensive and also states you don't know where you are going. You are not of a positive disposition and you are not speaking your truth or wanting or able to be heard. The neck is a continuation of the spinal column, so should be aligned as much as possible (so not head back either), but tension is frequently held in the neck and shoulders and head (migraine). Exposing the neck comes with increasing confidence. Once you have done so

you will be able to speak your truth and be more confident in being vulnerable.

Negativity
Let it go. It will hold you back and hold you down. If you hate someone or something it rebounds. Just let it go and leave room for creative stuff. You don't have to send out 'love' to someone you had hated a minute ago, but it's amazing if you try it; it releases you for so much positive stuff which has nothing to do with them or why you felt that negativity in the first place.

The same goes for if you feel negative about yourself. Ironically if you feel negative about yourself you are more inclined to feel negative about others (sometimes in the guise of jealousy or envy or pity). Feel positive about yourself and you'll find yourself feeling positive about others. Don't judge yourself or others.

Namaste

And peace be with you, Always say it at the end of class with your eyes closed. Do not open them for a few moments. Listen to your breath. Let peace be with you and in and around you.

O

OooMmmmm
Don't let everyone else say it. There are actually three vowels. Aaaaa, Ooooo Mmmmm. Say all of them. They show how your breath has developed at the end. Annunciate each in turn equally and see which one you fall 'short' on. Mmmm is usually the one – which symbolises love of self – Aaa (love of others, Ooo, love of earth, Mmmm love of self). Even the self-obsessed have difficulty with Mmm. Telling, huh?

Ojai
A town just outside California. It holds a yoga festival every October which takes over the place and offered everything from those in search of spiritual truth to those merely wanting to gain more flexibility and people watch, to those who run, spin, marathon, triathlete, iron man, and want to understand why they're doing it (me too).

P

Passion
What are you passionate about? Are you passionate about anything?

Try out a 'passion test' which identifies in a no nonsense way what is important to you. In a world where we want it all – it teaches you that you don't want it all. And what you do want will never be what you think. Its two sessions lasting between 75 to 90 minutes. Its empowering because you make the choices. It's time and money well spent. Accessible for both men and women, its pragmatic in approach, and will help you prioritise your life journeys – be they geographical or emotional. There's nothing grey about it – its black and white in your face life choices especially those of you who feel they lack direction (which is most of us do at one time or more in our lives).

I recommend having a one to one Passion Test with Jessica McGregor Johnson, International author, guide and coach, on Skype. Or you can also do the Passion Test in a workshop.

Jessica also offers individual and group retreats in Spain. www.jessicamcgregorjohnson.com/coaching.html   Or contact her direct on +44 (0) 203 239 6155 or jessica@jessicamcgregorjohnson.com

Private practice
A private session will cost you anything from £50 to £150 depending on the teacher you have, and probably more. It is more intensive and relentless but if you wish to perfect an asana or overcome one fear in a particular movement (head stand) it is worth making the investment. Continue with the group practice however, as the camaraderie of the class in yoga is worth it.

Pilates
When we breath in in yoga, they breath out in Pilates. When they breath out, in yoga we breath in. Pilates is exercise which stems from the logical working of the body. Yoga is a philosophy which stems from the need to find balance and focus in life. They are not alike, although they seem to be because both appear 'static'. The movements are static, and both are to do with in some way harnessing the breath, but they are from totally different planets. There's a T shirt which says 'yoga vs pilates'. It would be like saying apples vs meat balls.

Prayer
Meditation is a form of prayer. When you are practicing yoga, it is a form of prayer.

Q

Questions
Ask them, but preferably not at the end of the class but by text to the teacher afterwards. Take note of what you felt, the emotion during each asana and write it down. Then talk to the teacher about it, but not at the end of the class.

R

Reflect
How many of us take stock of how we are behaving. Learn how to. Contact Linda Linehan FCIPD, MBPS who

is a business coach but has an excellent technique on self reflection. www.abbevilleassociates.co.uk 020 7720 1830 mobile 07900 490465

Religion
One of the reasons I'm writing this book is because yoga has become very 'high church' and very Catholic in the way it's perceived. There is nothing great and good about doing a headstand for hours on end or being able to touch your bum with your head or vice versa. Yoga is accessible to everyone and should be communicated in a language everyone understands. Some will love the sanskrit, which is poetry, others will want to know how it will simply rid you of backache or headache or the pain in the left knee. It works, no matter what language you speak.

Running
Short bursts - 1/2 hour runs are best. Do not do long marathon type runs which age the skin. Practice yoga with either spinning or short runs and it produces a well balanced form of exercise regime.

Roots
Roots ground the tree. Look at your fingers when you are doing a downward dog. Space them out like roots. They give you grounding and support. Look after your hands, not just in a prettifying, painting nails way. But look at them and observe how you use them in and out of yoga. You will come to appreciate how they root you in everyday life.

S

Sahasrara Chakra – crown chakra
Located at the top of the head or the cerebral cortex, 'Sahasrara' means 'thousandfold'. Its colour is purple. A thousand lotus petals reside here. Its element is thought.

Its mantra is Aum or Om. Its function is to vitalise the brain.

Body parts it relates to include the pineal gland, cerebral cortex, central nervous system and right eye.

Balanced characteristics include the ability to analyse, perceive and assimilate information, intelligent, thoughtful and aware, open-minded, able to question, spiritually connected, wisdom with a broad understanding.

Negative characteristics include lack of inspiration, confusion, depression, hesitant to serve, learning difficulties, rigid belief system, apathy, an excess in the lower chakra (materialism, greed, or domination of others).

Physical effects include migraines, depression, amnesia, cognitive delusions.

Healing practices include meditation, learning and study, establishing a spiritual connection, examination of belief system.

Yoga poses which help include meditation, SAVASANA, UTTANASANA (standing forward fold), inversions SALAMBA SARVANGASANA (shoulder stand), PRASARITA PADOTTANASANA (standing wide leg forward fold), and ADHO MUKHA SVANASANA (downward facing dog).

Affirmations for this chakra are: The divine resides in me. I see myself and what I do with eyes of love. The world is my teacher. I am guided by inner wisdom. I am guided by a higher power.

Swadhisthana Chakra - Sacrum chakra

Located in the lower abdomen, close to the navel. The word 'Swadhisthana' means 'sweetness'. Its colour is orange. Six lotus petals reside here. Its element is water. Its Mantra is Vam. Its function is procreation, assimilation of food, source of sexuality, vitality and creativity.

The ovaries, testicles, prostate, genitals, spleen, womb and bladder relate to this chakra.

Balanced characteristics include graceful movements, emotional intelligence, ability to experience pleasure, nurturing of self and others, ability to change, and healthy boundaries.

Possible negative characteristics include poor boundaries with others, excessively strong emotions, overindulgence of food or sex, jealousy, envy, fear of change, frigidity or fear of sex, lack of passion, desire or excitement.

Physical impact includes impotency or sexual dysfunction, disorders of the reproductive organs, spleen, urinary system, lower back pain, and reduced flexibility.

Healing practices include movement therapy, emotional release or containment as appropriate, boundary work, inner child work, concentration on healthy pleasures.

Yoga postures which are good for this chakra include BADDHA KONASANA (bound ankle pose), JANU SIRSASANA (head to knee pose), SUPTA VIRASANA (reclining hero pose), ADHO MUKHA SVANASANA (downward facing dog), UTTANASANA (forward fold), UPAVISTHA KONASANA (seated wide leg pose), PRASARITA PADOTTANASANA (half moon pose), VIPARITA KARANI (legs up the wall pose).

Affirmations are: I accept my full power. I love and approve of myself. I am willing to change. I only create joyful experiences in my life. I deserve pleasure in my life. I move easily and effortlessly. Life is pleasurable.

Silence

Creating silence in your head is possible even when everything around you is noise. It's more important for you to do so when there is chaos around you. Being the calm in the storm, the eye in the middle of the hurricane, it happens when there is silence and stillness. Creating that stillness comes with practice through yoga. As you meditate, visualise yourself as an eagle soaring over hills and towns and villages, towards mountains, riding on the wind and against the storm, using the challenges to strengthen you. Feel the wind beneath your wings. This visualisation is about perspective. Rise above everything. When the wind pushes you in the opposite direction and there's a storm, treat it as a challenge. You have the strength to climb higher. Be the silence amongst the noise. Be the calm in the storm.

Strength
(emotional physical spiritual – I almost put this under P for power)We're talking inner strength as well as outer here and emotional, physical and mental. Breath and alignment help with clarity of thought, which in turn help you to identify what is needed, not just in yoga but in your other forms of exercise and lifestyle to gain and maintain strength.

Smile
Tyra Banks, supermodel and businesswoman, coined the phrase 'smizing': smiling with the eyes. You are able to smile with your whole body. Having that sense of joyfulness is created through practice of yoga. The eyes may be the window to the soul, but that joy should shine from every orifice of your body. The smile on the lips often masks an inner sadness. Yoga instructors look for posture, energy, tone of voice, not what the person is saying or if they are smiling. They look deeper.

Space
Create space in your mind. This happens during the Autumn, think September and children back to school. You need space to let new ideas generate. Think of the acorns growing into big oaks. This is the time of the acorn but in order to nurture these new ideas and act upon them you need to get rid of the old ideas and thoughts that are blocking you. Think how trees rid themselves of their leaves. Create space. Yoga helps you do this by focusing on your breath. Vinyasas are also excellent for creating a sense of space and clarity in the mind.

Sanskrit
Listening to Sanskrit is like listening to poetry - but if it detracts from knowing what to do next, it is obstructive. So it's all very well being high church and taking the class in sanskrit, but if no one knows what an uttanasana is and has to look at you and by the time they are in position you are onto a chataranga dandasana, then it's redundant. Sanskrit is the language of yoga, but should be gradually introduced to the class, unless you have a class that says, "Can we have this in sanskrit please?" I have done this with classes I have taught for a year and it works, but they still have to hesitate and look.

Shape
I interviewed Sir Terence Conran once, who told me that he designs furniture with an interest in what is around the space and how the space around his furniture is shaped. Think of the body that way. Look at the shapes you are creating around your movement and then you become less self-absorbed and conscious and more self-aware. The practice is very liberating.

Sun salutation
This is a series of six to seven moves at the beginning of a class, which activate all the chakras. They strengthen the core, improve alignment and flexibility, focus the mind and deepen the breath; in short, it is a wonderful way to start the class. There have been classes where the series of sun salutations have been introduced throughout the class exclusively. So after an hour, you will have completed a hundred. You will be sweating and exhilarated.

Shoulder stand
For those wanting to attempt more challenging inversions this is an excellent way to start out. Shoulder stands work all the chakras and are particularly good for suppressing appetite, alleviating stress, focusing the mind, improving

circulation and good for depression and memory loss. Try to stay up there for 18 seconds (slow count) and keep the elbows close together (hold the elbows with the hands and keep them in position). You will be able to lift and straighten your torso more effectively and maintain the posture for longer. An excellent way to end a class before svanasana or fish pose.

Spirit
Small word, big meaning. I am frequently told I'm a free spirit. It is more a state of mind than anything. You are always a 'non fitter inner' but don't shout about it. It's a bit like saying you're interesting or different. If you are interesting and different other people tell you you are. Or they don't, because they feel nervous around you (people who don't understand you, will fear you – it's a very English thing rather than a very human thing). Having a positive, vibrant spirit is what life is about. You are a spirit with a body not a body with a spirit. Basically, it's what makes you you. Combined with what you look like, how you identify with others, how you learn (or don't learn), but it's your ability to stand back and, like the child in 'The Emperor with no clothes' say, 'I choose'. That's spirit. Of course there's also lost spirits, who have essentially lost all sense of value and perspective and self-awareness. People frequently come to yoga to bolster their spirit – they just call it confidence, but spirit is essentially what it is.

T

Thoughts
I started yoga because my head was always buzzing with ideas, characters, new books, new initiatives, which I either half started or didn't really think through. Yoga helped to focus and clear my mind and it took till my forties to appreciate that and really to get the full benefit from it. The more life experience you have, the more you need to file

away and create space for yourself. When you're in your twenties it's all about the flexibility, and focusing on the body, when you're in your forties, it's about having that sense of embodiment but being aware how it talks to you and tells you what is both right and wrong in your life. The mind plays tricks on us, telling us things which are not true. The body never lies. Yoga teaches you how to listen to your body, and connect with it.

Trikonasana
Triangle pose works all chakras, but especially the heart, throat and solar plexus, rooting us. It has variations but it opens us up to the sky, releasing tensions and blockages in our bodies, and strengthening our breath in the process.

Trends
Yoga has trends like everything else. Dynamic yoga, power, hatha, iyengar, vinyasa, ashtanga, there are so many. Try them all, they complement each other. Also try out and combine other forms of exercise. I don't suggest you do yoga and nothing else. Go spinning, run for fifteen minutes and no more than half an hour or dance. Yoga is part of the jigsaw puzzle along with eating healthily, so treat it that way. Don't be afraid to try something new. Yoga will help you overcome fear of trying something new.

Tums
Abdominals. Flat tummies, hard bodies were in in the 70s and 80s. Having a little tummy is sexy. Not a big one, a little one. Upward and downward dogs are wonderful for the abdominals. You will find the sun salutation works the tum more than any stomach crunches could, as well as other parts of the body.

Thighs
How to get rid of flabby upper thighs. Yoga provides balance in the mind and body and so it will in the body. A

combination of running and spinning along with yoga and dance classes (modern jazz is best) will help with this area. Focus on lengthening the area rather than building it up. So keep the running and spinning short. Dance as much as you want to.

Teachers
Find one that works for you and continue to try out new ones. Find one that is local. If you find a great one you need to travel an hour for, weigh up the pros and cons. And just because your friend clicks with a teacher doesn't mean you will. Take note of that.

Time
Classes range from an hour to hour and a half. Private practice for half an hour each morning is fine, even less. But find time to practice each morning. It will be worth it to set up the day and focus your mind.

Trees
Was almost not going to put this in, but a tree is used so often in visualisation, in meditation - the tree pose in yoga is one of the most stabilising and strengthening. Uplifting and grounding at the same time, it makes us aware of what we are capable of - literally reaching out in both directions. Trees are wonderful things. Go hug one next time you are on a jog/walk.

Truth
Find it. At least try to.

U

Upside down (or inversions)
Inversions create fear in a lot of people. Realise this and invest in a private session to get over the fear as inversions are very good for dealing with stress and empowerment.

V

Visshuddha Chakra - throat chakra
Located at the throat centre. 'Visshuddha' means' purification'. Its colour is sky blue. Six lotus petals are located here. Its element is sound. Its Mantra is Ham. Its function is speech, sound vibration, creativity, listening and communication.

Body parts relate to thyroid, parathyroid, hypothalamus, throat and mouth.

Balanced characteristics include resonant voice, good listener, good sense of timing and rhythm, clear communication skills, truthful, expressive, living creatively.

Negative characteristics include fear of speaking, difficulty putting feelings to words, small weak voice, shyness, poor rhythm, tone deaf, gossips, too much talking, inability to listen, interrupting, dominating voice.

Physical malfunctions include disorders of the throat, ears, voice, neck, tight jaw, stiff neck and toxicity.

Yoga poses which are good for the throat chakra include SIMHASANA (lions pose), MATSYASANA (fish pose), PARSVOTTANASANA (intense side stretch), JATHARA PARIVARTANASANA (supine twist or bent knee twist), USTRASANA (camel pose), SETU BANDHA SARVANGASANA (bridge pose), ADHO MUKHA SVANASANA (downward facing dog) BHUJANGASANA (cobra pose) VIRABHADRASANA II (Warrior II)

Affirmations include: I am willing to change. I express myself freely and joyously. Divine ideas are expressed through me. It is safe to see other viewpoints. Creativity flows in and through me. I hear and speak the truth. My voice is necessary.

Voice
Speaking your truth. The Visshuddha chakra, finding your voice. The English culture is to look down, hide the

neck, be closed in, and keep things to yourself. Yoga is about opening up and releasing tensions that restrict our mental, emotional and spiritual growth. Speaking your truth is a powerful way to achieve this.

Vision board
Go to an art shop and buy a large A3 or bigger size of white card. Get magazines. Cut out words and photos that symbolise where you want to be. Your inspiration as well as your aspiration. I chose mountains and sunshine and Tom and me and Indian chiefs, and hummingbirds (they are the only birds who can fly backwards as well as forwards to get what they want) and me on the front cover of a magazine with the words 'crusading pilot'. Yup. Do your own and put it on your bedroom wall behind you and see where it takes you. Better than a top ten of what you want to achieve each year.

Vinyasa
'Vinyasa' means flow. So vinyasa flow is 'flow flow' yoga. It is a series of sun salutations which generate heat in the body, regulate breath, strengthen the core, lengthen the hamstrings and spine, open the chest and work all the chakras. In short, it is a wonderful way to start a yoga practice or even be the main constituent of it. Forget the stomach crunches. This series of movements works the abdominals.

W

Weight
It doesn't matter how much you weigh, although it does impact on what postures you are actually able to get into.

CHAPTER FIVE

TEN MINUTE YOGA SEQUENCE FOR EMOTIONAL BAGGAGE

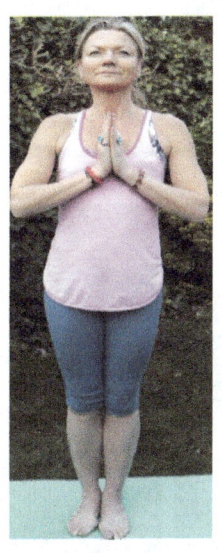

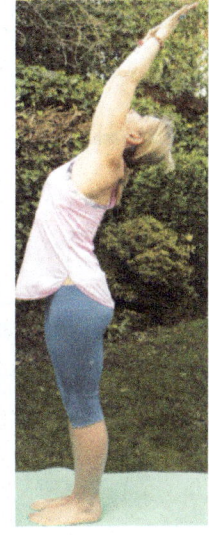

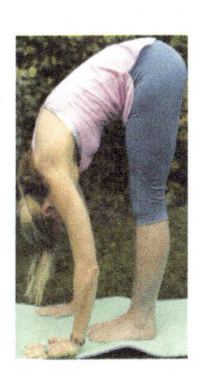

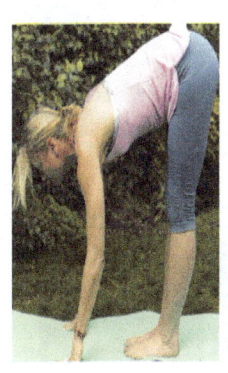

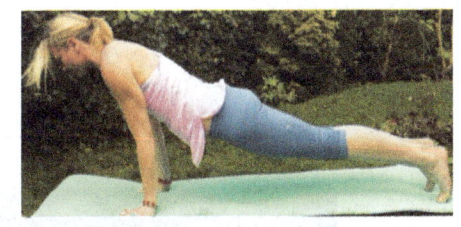

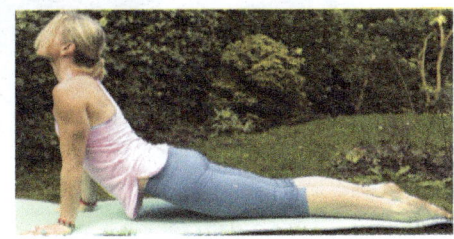

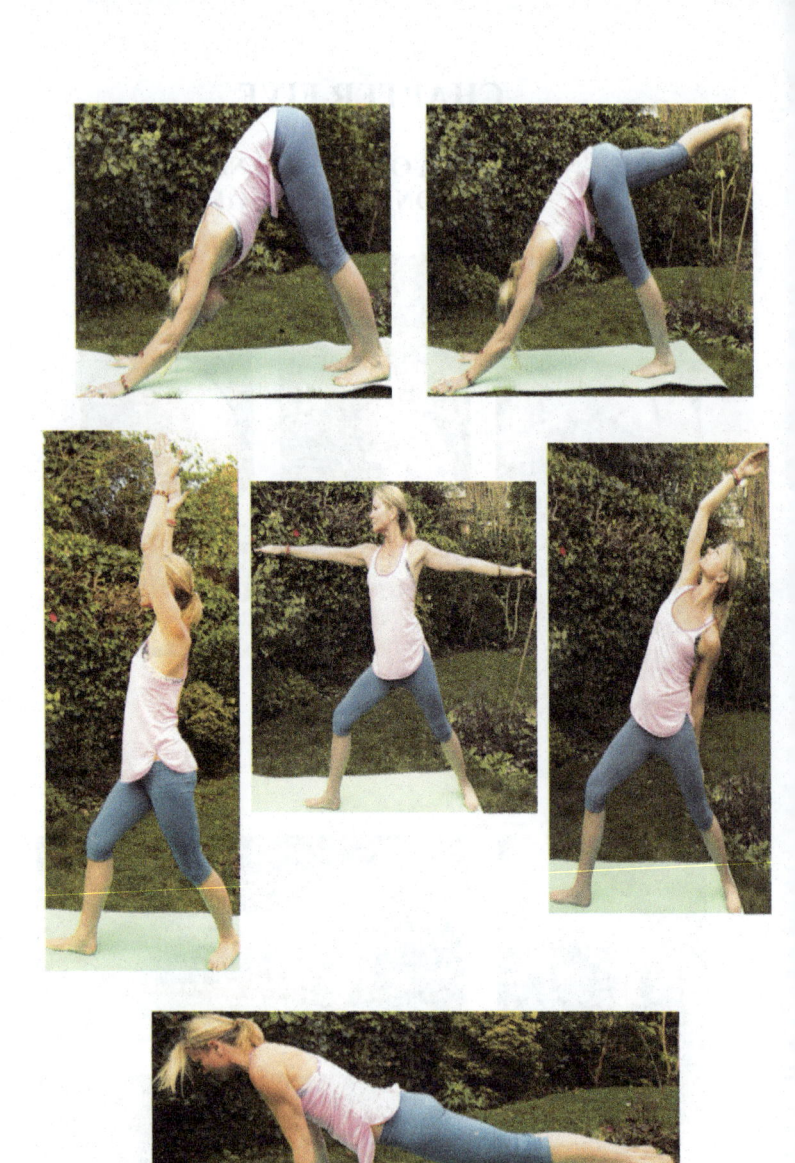

Music (if appropriate) Yoga Sessions by Go Ray and Duke

SHAKTI NAMASKAR 5 minutes

Stand in tadasana, shoulders back, head up as if being pulled by a piece of golden thread.

INHALE	Rise on balls of the feet, arms overhead in prayer, look up
EXHALE	Tadasana, heels to earth, palms to chest
INHALE	Hook tubs, reach up and arch back
EXHALE	Uttanasana, fold forward bend
INHALE	Ardha uttanasana, look up
EXHALE	Step or jump back to Chaturanga dandasana
INHALE	Urdhva mukha svanasana, upward dog, relax shoulders
EXHALE	Adho mukha svanasana, hold for three breaths. Breath in, through the nose. Stretch out that back, keeping the hips and back straight. Palms of the hands flat on the floor. Fingers stretched out. Relax the shoulders. Use the strength of your arms and legs to fully and evenly stretch your spine. Stretch your hips, hamstrings and calves. This posture strengthens your quadriceps and ankles. Opens your chest and shoulders, tones your arms and abdominals. Even tones your hands and feet.
INHALE	Ardha uttanasana, jump or step forward, look up
EXHALE	Fold uttanasana
INHALE	Urdhva hastasana, reach up, arms shoulder width apart, palms facing each other.
EXHALE	Tadasana, hands to chest Repeat two to four times. If you feel at any time you need to break, just move into child's pose.

SURYA NAMASKAR 5 MINS

INHALE	Bend knees into chair. Utkatasana
EXHALE	Fold uttanasana
INHALE	Ardha uttanasana
EXHALE	Step or jump back, chataranga dandasana
INHALE	Upward dog, urdhva mukha svanasana
EXHALE	Downward dog, adho mukha svanasana
INHALE	Right leg raise ska pads mukha svanasana, keep hips square.
EXHALE	Step right foot forward and keep the back heel down
INHALE	Warrior One Virabhadrasana Eki; this is a strong pose, warrior pose, feel like a warrior.
EXHALE	Warrior Two Virabhadrasana Dvi
INHALE	Reverse Warrior
EXHALE	hands to floor, chaturanga dandasana
INHALE	upward dog, urdhva mukha svanasana
	EXHALE downward dog, adho mukha svanasana. Hold for three breaths. Keep the tension neck.
INHALE	Ardha uttanasana, jump forward look up
EXHALE	Fold uttanasana
INHALE	Utkatasana
EXHALE	Tadasana, hands in prayer
INHALE	Bend knees chair, Utkatasana
EXHALE	Fold uttanasana
INHALE	Ardha uttanasana
EXHALE	Chataranga dandasana
INHALE	Left leg raise ska pads mukha svanasana, keep hips square
EXHALE	Step left foot forward and keep the back heel down
INHALE	Warrior One, Virabhadrasana Eki, this is a strong pose, warrior pose, strong through

	the arms and legs, both feet rooted. Phalakasana.
EXHALE	Warrior Two Virabhadrasana Dvi
INHALE	Reverse Warrior
EXHALE	Hands to floor, chaturanga dandasana
INHALE	Upward dog, urdhva mukha svanasana
EXHALE	Downward dog, adho mukha savasana. Hold for three breaths. Keep the position strong.
	Feel the stretch through the back, shoulders relaxed. Keep the tension out of the shoulders. Head down. Relax the neck.
INHALE	Ardha uttanasana, jump forward and look up
EXHALE	Fold uttanasana
INHALE	Utkatasana
EXHALE	Tadasana, hands in prayer

CHAPTER SIX

YOGA POSE DIRECTORY IN SANSKRIT / ENGLISH

A

Adho Mukha Baddha Kona Utthita Vrschikasana
 Downward Facing Bound Feet Elevated Scorpion Pose
Adho Mukha Ekapada Sirsa Bakasana
 One-Foot Behind The Head Downward Facing Crane Pose
Adho Mukha Mandukasana
 Downward Facing Frog
Adhomukha Parivrrtapada Baddha Konasana
 Downward Facing Twisted Feet Bound
Adho Mukha Svanasana
 Downward Facing Dog
Adho Mukha Vrksasana
 Downward Facing Tree Pose Handstand Prep.
Adho Mukha Vrksasana
 Downward Facing Tree Pose/ Hand Stand
Agasthiy Arasana
 Sage Agasthiyar Pose
Agnistambhasana
 Firelog
Akarna Dhanurasana
 Shooting Bow Pose
Akarna Dhanurasana I
 Archer Pose I
Akarna Dhanurasana II
 Archer Pose II (Var.)
Alamba Bhujangasana
 Supported Cobra Pose
Alamba Urdhva Paschimottanasana
 Supported Upward Tending Intense Back Stretch Pose
Alamba Vygarasana
 Supported Tiger stretch Pose

Ananda Balasana
　Joyful Baby
Ananda Paksiyasana
　Happy Bird Pose
Anantasana I
　Infinity Pose
Anantasana II
　Reclining Pose Dedicated to Vishnu
Andar Mukha Pinchapada Sirsasana
　Face Under The Body Foot Behind The Head Chin Lock Pose
Andar Mukha Prasarita Padotanasana
　Face Under The Body Wide Legs Forward bend Pose
Andar Mukha Viparita Dwi Pada Dandasana
　Face in Between The Legs Full backbend Staff Pose
Andiappan Asana
　Yogi Andiappan Pose
Anuvittasana
　Standing Backbend
Araniasana
　Dragon Pose
Ardha Agasthiyar Asana
　Sage Agasthiyar Pose – Half
Ardha-Baddha Padma Paschimatanasana
　Half-Bound Lotus Back Stretch Pose
Ardha Baddha Padma Padangustha Sirsanasa
　Bound Half Lotus – Head to Big Toe Pose
Ardha Baddha Padma Padangusthasana
　Bound Half Lotus Tiptoe Pose
Ardha Baddha Padma Padangusthasana
　Bound Half Lotus Tiptoe Pose
Ardha Baddha Padma Paschimatanasana
　Half-Bound Lotus Forward Bend
Ardha Baddha Padma Prapardasana
　Half-Bound Lotus Tiptoe Pose
Ardha Baddha Padma Setu Bandhasana
　Bound Half Lotus Bridge Pose
Ardha Padma Baddha Utkatasana

  Bound Half Lotus Powerful Pose
Ardha Baddha Setu Bandhasana
  Half Bound Lotus Bridge-Forming Pose
Ardha Baddha Padmottanasana
  Half Bound Lotus Intense Stretch Pose
Ardha Bakasana
  Crane Pose – Half
Ardha Bogarasana
  Sage Bogar Pose – Half
Ardha Chandrasana
  Half Moon Pose Prep
Ardha Chandrasana
  Half Moon Pose
Ardha Gomukha Paschimottanasana
  Half Cow Face Forward Bend
Ardha Kamalamuniasana
  Sage Kamalamuniasana Pose – Half
Ardha Mandalasana
  Half Circle
Ardha Matsyasana
  Half Fish Pose
Ardha Matsyendrasana
  Sage Matsyendra Pose (Half)
Ardha Matsyendrasana
  Half Lord of the Fishes Pose
Ardha Namaskar Parsvakonasana
  Half Prayer Twist
Ardha Navasana
  Half Boat Pose
Ardha Padangustha Himalaryasana
  One Arm Holding The Big Toe – Mount Himalaya Pose – Half
Ardha Padma Adho Mukha Vrksasana
  Half Lotus in Handstand
Ardha Padma Baddha
  Bound Half Lotus Tiptoe Balancing Pose
Ardha Padma Baddha Padangusthasana
  Bound Half Lotus Tiptoe Balancing Pose

Ardha Padma Eka Pada Padmottanasana
  Half Lotus One Leg Stretched Up Pose
Ardha Padmasana
  Half-Lotus Pose
Ardha Padmasana in Vrksasana
  Tree Pose in Half Lotus
Ardha Parsva Konasana
  Side Angle Pose – Half
Ardha Parsvottanasana
  Half Pyramid
Ardha Pasasana
  Noose Pose – Half
Ardha Pavana Muktasana
  Half Wind Relieving Pose
Ardha Phalakasana
  Low Plank
Ardha Pincha Mayurasana
  Dolphin
Ardha Salamba-Shirshasana
  Supported Half Head Stand Pose
Ardha Sarvangasana
  Half Shoulder Stand Pose
Ardha Shalabhasana
  Half Locust Pose
Ardha Shirshasana
  Half Head Pose
Ardha Shalabhasana
  Half Locust Pose
Ardha Supta Virasana
  Half Supine Hero
Ardha Ustrasana
  Camel Pose – Half
Ardha Utripada Sirsasna
  Tripod Headstand Pose – Half
Ardha Uttanasana
  Half Standing Forward Bend
Ardha Urdhva Upavishta Konasana
  Half Upright Seated Angle

Ardha Ustrasana
  Half Camel Pose
Ardha-Vayu-Muktyasana
  Half Wind-Relieving Pose
Ardha Virabhadrasana I
  Low Warrior I
Ardha Vrschikasana
  Half Scorpion Pose
Arjunasana
  Prince Arjuna Pose
Ashtangasana
  Eight-Limbed Pose
Ashwa Sanchalanasana
  Equestrian Pose
Asta Vakrasana
  Balance Dedicated to Astavakra/Eight Twists Pose
Atirupa Mayurasana
  Beautiful Peacock Pose
Avakra Vrschikasana
  Upright Scorpion Pose

B

Baddha Akarna Dhanurasana
  Bound Archer Pose
Baddha Hastha Dwipada Viparita Dandasana
  Bound Arms Both Legs Inverted Staff Pose
Baddha Hasta Padma Shirshasana/Sirsasana
  Bound Arms Lotus Headstand Pose
Baddha Hastha Parivrtta Parsva Konasana
  Bound Arms Revolved Side Angle Pose
Baddha Hastha Parsva Konasana
  Bound Arms Angle Pose
Baddha Hasta Shirshasana/Sirsasana
  Bound Hand Headstand
Baddha Hastha Utthita Eka Pada Viparita Dandasana
  Bound Arms One Leg Stretched Up Inverted staff Pose

Baddha Konasana
  Bound Angle Pose/Cobbler Pose
Baddha Konasana in Niralamba Sirsasana
  Bound Angle Unsupported Headstand
Baddha Konasana in Sarvangasana
  Bound Angle Shoulder Stand I
Baddha Konasana in Sirsasana I
  Bound Angle Headstand I
Baddha Matsyasana
  Bound Fish Pose
Baddha Natarajasana
  Bound Lord of the Dance Pose
Baddha Pada Ardha Padma Vrschikasana
  Bound Foot Half Lotus Scorpion Pose
Baddha Pada Mastyasana
  Bound Legs Fish Pose
Baddha Pada Parivrtta Konasana
  Bound Leg Twisted Triangle Pose
Baddha Padmasana
  Bound Lotus Pose
Baddha Padmottanasana
  Locked Elbow Standing Forward Bend Pose
Baddha Pada Nirlamba Sarvangasana
  Bound Feet – -Unsupported Whole Body Rejuvenating Pose
Baddha Pada Viparita Dandasana
  Bound Foot Inverted staff Pose
Baddha Yajnasana
  Bound Christ's Cross Pose
Baddhapada Akarna Dhanurasana
  Bound Leg Archer Pose
Baddhapada Koormamuni Asana
  Bound Legs Sage Koormamuni Pose
Bakasana
  Crane Pose
Balancing Table
Balasana
  Child Pose

Bhadrasana
  Gracious Pose
Bhairavasana
  Reclining Formidable Pose
Bharadvajasana I
  Twist Dedicated to Bharadvajra
Bharadvajasana II
  Twist Dedicated to Bharadvajra II
Bhekasana
  Frog Pose
Bhadrasana
  Gracious Pose
Bhairavasana
  Formidable Shiva Pose
Bharadvajasana
  Pose of the Sage Warrior Bharadvaja
Bhujapidasana
  Shoulder Pressing Arm Balance
Bhujangasna I
  Cobra Pose
Bhujangasna II
  Cobra Pose
Bhujangasna III
  Cobra Pose
Bhujamadya Sirsa Samakonasana
  Elbow Supported Headstand Same Angle Pose
Bhujamadya Padma Sirsasana
  Elbow Supported Headstand Pose
Bhramariasana
  Honeybee Pose
Bhujangasana
  Cobra Pose
Bhunamanasana
  Saluting Mother Earth Pose
Bogar
  Sage Pose Forward BendIng
Brahmacharyasana
  Celebate Pose

Bramhamuniasana
  Sage Bramhamuni Pose
Buddhasana
  Enlightened Pose

C

Chakorasana
  Moonbird Pose
Chakorasana
  Partridge Pose
Chakorasana
  Partridge Pose
Chakorasana
  Moon Bird Pose
Chakra Bandasana
  Bound Wheel Pose
Chakrasana
  Wheel Pose
Chandrasana
  Crescent Moon
Chaturanga
  Four Limbed Staff Pose
Chaturanga Dandasana
  Four-Limbed staff Pose
Chatuskonasana
  Four Corner Pose
Catuspadapitham
  Crab Pose
Chalanasana
  Churning Pose

D

Dandasana
  Staff Pose
Dakshina Nauli
  Right Side Isolation

Dandayamna Baddha Konasana
  Balancing Bound Angle
Dandayamana Janu Sirsasana
  Standing Head To Knee
Dandayamana Yoga Mudrasana
  Standing Yoga Seal
Dandayamna Baddha Konasana
  Balancing Bound Angle
Dhanurasana
  Bow Pose
Dur Dhanurasana
  Difficult Bow Pose
Durvasanana/Durvasana
  Pose of the Sage Durva
Durvasana
  Pose of the Sage Durva (Preparation)
Dwi Hasta Bhujasana
  Two-Handed Arm Balance
Dwi-Pada-Anantasana
  Two-Leg Infinity Pose
Dwi-Pada-Koundinyasana
  Two-Legged Arm Balance of the Sage Koundinya
Dwi Pada Sirsasana
  Two-Feet-Behind-the-Head Pose/Balancing Tortoise Pose
Dwi Pada Viparita
  Two-Legged Inverted
Dwi Pada Viparita Dandasana
  Two-Legged Inverted Staff Pose
Dwi Pada Yoga Dandasana
  Yogi's Meditation stick Pose/Two-Legged Yogi Staff Balance

E

Edaikaadar Asana
  Sage Edailaadar Pose

Eka Hasta Adho Mukha Vrkshasana
  One-Hand Hand stand Pose
Eka Hasta Bhujasana
  One-Leg-Arm Balance
Eka Hasta Korarasana
  One Arm Raised Up Sage Koarkar Pose
Eka Hasta Padagustha Naukasana
  One Arm Holding The Big Toe Boat Pose
Eka Hasta Padapaschima Rajakapotasana
  Feet Touching The Back King Pigeon – One Arm
Eka Hasta Padma Sirsasana
  One Arm Balance – Lotus Headstand Pose
Eka Hasta Padma Mayurasana
  One Arm Balance Lotus Peacock Pose
Eka Hasta Padma Adho-Mukha-Vrkshasana
  One-Hand Lotus Hand Stand Pose
Eka Hasta Paripurna Hanumanasana
  One Arm Lord Hanuman Pose – Complete
Eka Hasta Parivid Pada Dhanurasana
  Twined Legs Bow Pose – One Arm
Eka Hasta Parsva Padma Sarvangasana
  Sideways Upward Tending Lotus In Whole Body
  Rejuvenating Pose With One
Eka Hasta Parsva Padma Sarvangasana
  Sideways Upward Tending Lotus in Padma
Sethubandhasana
  Whole Body Rejuvenating Pose With One Arm Balance
Eka Hasta Prasarita Apda Sirsasana
  Feet Spread Out One Arm Balance Headstand Pose
Eka Hasta Purvottanasana
  Single Arm Intense Front Body Stretch Pose
Eka Hasta Sivanandasana
  Yogi Sivananda Pose – One Arm Variation
Eka Hasta Thirumoolarasana
  One Arm Balance Sage Thirumoolar Pose
Eka Hasta Tirianf Mukhttona Natarjasana
  Intense Backbend Shiva's Dancing Pose

Eka Hasta Urdhvamukha Paripruna Nindra Nindra Dhanurasana
  Upward Facing One Arm at Standing Full Bow Pulling Pose
Eka Hasta Vyaghrasana
  One Handed Tiger
Eka Hasta Adho Mukha Vrksasana
  One Hand Handstand Pose
Eka Pada Adho Muckha Svanasana
  One-Legged Downward Facing Dog Pose
Eka Pada Adho Mukha Svanasana
  One Leg Downward Facing Dog
Eka Pada Baddha Galavasana
  Bound Lef Sage Galava Pose
Eka Pada Badha Hasta Uttanasana
  One Leg Hand Binding Intense Stretch Pose
Eka Pada Baddha Paripurna Veerasana
  Bound Foot Complete Warrior Pose
Eka Pada Baddha Utthita Vrschikasana
  Bound Foot Elevated Scorpion Pose
Eka Pada Baddha Veerasana
  Bound Foot Warrior Pose
Eka Pada Baddha Vrschikasana
  Bound Foot Scorpion Pose
Eka Pada Bakasana
  One-Legged Crane Pose
Eka-Pada Dhanurasana
  One Leg Bow Pose
Eka Pada Eka Hasta Rajpotasana
  One Arm and One Leg King Pigeon Pose
Eka Pada Galavasana
  One-Legged Balance Sage Galava Pose
Eka Hasta Shirshasana
  One Hand Head Stand Pose (Reverse Hand Var.)
Eka Pada Vasisthasana
  One Arm Holding the Big Toe Sage Vasistha
Eka Hasta Vyaghrasana
  One Handed Tiger

Eka Pada Kapatosana
  One-Leg Pigeon Pose
Eka Pada Koundinyasana
  One Leg Sage Koundinya Pose
Eka-Pada-Niralamba-Shirshasana
  One Foot Hands-Free Head Stand Pose
Eka Pada Padangustha Dhanurasna
  One-Legged Big-Toe Bow Pose
Eka Pada Koundinyasana I
  One-Legged Arm Balance for Koundinyasana I
Eka Pada Koundinyasana II
  One-Legged Arm Balance for Koundinyasana II
Eka Pada Konganarasana
  Sage Konganar Pose – One Leg
Eka Pada Mukta Hasta Sirsasana
  One-Legged Free-Hand Headstand
Eka Pada Navasana
  One-Legged Boat Pose
Eka Pada Nikunjasana
  One Leg Raised Heart
Eka Pada Nindra Rajakapotasana
  One Leg King Pigeon Pose
Eka Padangustha Vasisthasana
  Balance Dedicated to the Sage Vasistha
Eka Padangustha Vyaghrasana
  One Arm Holding The BigToe Tiger Stretch Pose
Eka-Pada-Raja-Bhujangasana
  One-Leg King Cobra Pose
Eka Pada Rajakapotasana I
  One-Legged King Pigeon Pose
Eka Pada Rajakapotasana II
  One-Legged King Pigeon Pose II
Eka Pada Salamba-Shirshasana
  Supported One-Leg Head stand Pose
Eka Pada Sarvangasana
  One-Legged Shoulder Stand I
Eka Pada Setubandha Sarvangasana
  One Leg Stretched Up Bridge Pose

Eka Pada Setu Bandhasana
  One-Legged Bridge Pose
Eka Pada Setu Bandha Sarvangasana
  One-Legged Bridge Pose
Eka Pada Shirsha Rajakapotasana
  One Leg to Head Pigeon Pose
Eka Pada Shirshasana
  One Leg Behind the Head Pose
Eka Pada Sirsasana
  Foot Behind The Head Pose
Eka Pada Sirsasana I
  One-Legged Headstand I
Eka Pada Sirsa Ananda Sayanasana
  Foot Behind The Head Yogi's Resting Pose
Eka Pada Sirsa Bakasana
  One-Foot-Behind-the-Head Crane Pose
Eka Pada Sirsa Nirakunjasana
  Foot To Head Heart Pose
Eka Pada Sirsa Padangusthasana
  Foot-Behind-the-Head-Tip-Toe Pose
Eka Pada Sirsa Yoga Dandasana
  Foot Behind The Head In Yogi's Meditating Stick Pose
  Extended Leg Squat
Eka Pada Urdhva Adomukha Svanasana
  One Leg Raised Up Downward Facing Dog Pose
Eka Pada Urdhva Dhanurasana
  One-Legged Inverted Bow Pose
Eka Pada Utthana Mercudhandasana
  One Leg Stretched Up Intense Backbend Pose
Eka Pada Vasisthasana
  One Leg Sage Vasistha Pose
Eka Pada Viparita Dandasana
  One Leg Inverted Staff Pose
Eka Pada Viparita Dandasana
  One Leg Inverted Staff Pose
Eka Pada ViparitaDandasana I
  One Leg Inverted Staff Pose I

Eka Pada ViparitaDandasana I
  One Leg Inverted Staff Pose I (Var.)
Eka Pada Viparita Dandasana I
  One-Legged Inverted Staff Pose
Eka Pada Viparita Dandasana I
  One-Legged Inverted Staff Pose
Eka Pada ViparitaDandasana II
  One Leg Inverted Staff Pose II
Eka Pada Viparita Dandasana II
  One-Legged Inverted Staff Pose II
Eka Pada Viparita Dandasana II
  One-Legged Inverted Staff Pose II
Eka Pada Vrschikasana
  One-Leg Scorpion Pose
Eka Pada Vrschikasana II
  One-Legged Scorpion Pose
Eka Pada Yoganidrasana
  Yogi's Sleeping Pose
Eka Padaya Paripurna Vrschikasana
  One Leg Stretched Out Lotus In Scorpion Pose

F

Flowering Lotus

G

Gaivasana
  Chain Pose
Galavasana
  Pose of the Sage Galava
Ganda Bherundasana
  Formidable Face Pose
Garbha Pindasana
  Embryo /Baby in The Womb Pose
Garudasana
  Eagle Pose

Garudasana in Adho Mukha Vrksasana
  Eagle Pose in Handstand
Garudasana in Sarvangasana I
  Shoulder Stand with Eagle Legs I
Garudasana in Sirsasana I
  Headstand with eagle Legs I
Gheransasana
  Pose Dedicated to the Sage Gheranda
Gitanandasana
  Yogi Gitananda Pose
Gomukhasana
  Cow Face Pose
Goraksasana
  Pose of the Lord Goraksha /Sage Goraksa /Cowherd Pose
Garbhasana
  Child's Pose
Gupta Padmasana
  Hidden Lotus Pose

H

Halasana
  Plough Pose
Hansasana
  Swan Pose
Hanumanasana
  Pose of the Lord Hanuman/Leg-Split Pose
Hanumanasana in Adho Mukha Vrksasana
  Split Legs in Handstand
Hanumanasana Sirsasana I
  Headstand with Front Splits Headstand I
Hanumanasana Namaskara
  Hanuman Salutation Pose
Hanumanasana Pincha Mayurasana
  Split Legs in Peacock Feather Pose
Himalayasana
  Mount Himalaya Pose

I

Iyengar Asana
  Yogi Iyengar Pose

J

Jalandhara Bandha
  Chin Lock dm647
Janu Sirsasana/ Shirshasana
  Head-to-Knee Pose
Janu Sirsa Brahmacharyasana
  Head To Knee Celebate Pose
Jathara Parivartanasana
  Twisted Stomach Pose
Jatharasana
  Abdominal Lift Pose

K

Kailiasana
  Goddess Kali Pose
Kailashasana
  Lord Kaliasha Pose
Kakasana
  Crow Pose
Kala Bhairavasana
  Balance Dedicated to the Universal Destroyer Shiva
Kamalamuni
  Asana Sage Kamalamuni Pose
Kamalasana
  Goddess Kamala Pose
Kandasana
  Navel Pose
Kandharasana
  Shoulder Pose
Kanjanasana
  Wagtail Pose

Kapinjalasana
  Partridge Pose
Kapinjalasana
  Raindrop-Drinking Bird Pose
Kapinjalasana
  Raindrop-Drinking Bird Pose
Kapinjalasana
  Partridge Pose
Kapotasana
  Pigeon Pose
Kapyasana
  Monkey Pose
Karandavasana
  Duck Pose
Karnapidasana
  Ear Pressure Pose/ Knee to Ear Pose
Karnapida Chakrasana
  Ear Pressure Wheel Pose
Kashyapasana
  Pose of the Sage Kashyapa
Konasana Chikka
  Asana Book Stand Pose
Konganarasana
  Sage Konganar Pose
Koormamuni
  Sage Koormamuni Pose
Koormasana
  Tortoise Pose
Korakarasana
  Sage Korakar Pose
Koundinyasana
  Sage Koundinya Pose
Krounchasana
  Heron Pose
Kukkutasana
  Cock Pose
Kulphasana
  Ankle Pose

Kulpha-Vrkshasana
  Ankle Tree Pose
Kulpha-Vrkshasana
  Ankle Tree Pose (Var One Arm Up)
Kulpha Vrkshasana
  Ankle Tree Pose (Var Hand on Hip)
Kuntasana
  Spear Pose
Kunthasana
  Full Squat Pose

L

Leg Cradle
  Laghu Chakrasana
Little Wheel Pose
  Laghu Dhanurasana
Little Bow Pose
  Laghu Vajrasana
Little/ Graceful Thunderbolt Pose
  Lingasana Shivalinga Pose
Lolasana
  Pendulum/ Pendant/ Dangling Pose

M

Madyama Nauli
  Central Abdominal Contraction
Maha Mudra
  The Great Seal / Powerful Seal
Makarasana
  Crocodile Pose
Malasana
  Garland Pose
Mandalasana Parampara
  Circle Pose Series
Mandukasana
  Frog Pose

Marjaryasana
  Cat stretch Pose
Matsyasana
  Fish Pose
Mayurasana
  Peacock Pose
Marichyasana I
  Dedicated to Sage Marichi
Marichyasana II
  Dedicated to Sage Marichi II
Marichyasana III
  Dedicated to Sage Marichi III
Marichyasana IV
  Dedicated to Sage Marichi IV
Moola Bhandasana
  Root Lock/ Perineal Contraction Pose
Moola Matsyendrasana
  Sage Matsyendra Pose
Mukta Hasta Sirsasana
  Free-Hand Headstand
Mulabandhasana
  Root Chakra/ Lock Pose
Musti Purvottanasana
  Intense Front Body Stretch Pose
Musti Padma Mayurasana
  Fist Lotus Peacock Pose

N

Nadi Vibrator-Pranayama
Nartana Mayurasana
  Dancing Peacock Pose
Natarajasana
  Lord of the Dance Pose
Natarajasana
  Dancer's Pose (Variation Changed From Prep)
Natarajasana I
  Lord of the Dance Pose I

Natarajasana
 Dancer's Pose (Variation to Prep)
Natarajasana
 Lord of the Dance Pose
Natarajasana
 Dancer's Pose (Variation)
Natarajasana
 Dancer's Pose (Variation)
Natarajasana
 Dancer's Pose (Variation)
Natarajasana
 Dancer's Pose (Variation)
Natarajasana
 Ballet Pose (Variation)
Natarajasana II
 Lord of the Dance Pose II
Niralamba Sirsasana I
 Unsupported Headstand Arms & Legs Spread Wide
Niralamba Sirsasana II
 Unsupported Headstand
Namaskar Parsvakonasana
 Prayer Twist
Namaskarasana
 Prayer Squat
Nandiasana
 Lord Nandi Pose
Natyasana
 Ballet Pose
Naukasana
 Boat Pose
Navasana
 Boat Pose
Nindra Vayu Mukttonasana
 Standing Wind Releasing Forward Bend Pose
Nindra Vayu Muktyasana
 Standing Wind Releasing Pose
Nindra Ananda Paksiyasana
 Standing Happy Bird Pose

Nindra Rajapotasana
  Standing King Pigeon Pose
Nindra Valakhilasana
  Divine Spirit Pose
Nirakunjasana
  Heart Pose
Nirlamba Baddha Eka Pada Uttanasana
  Unsupported Bound Foot Forward Bend Pose
Nirlamba Paripurna Bhujangasana
  Unsupported Cobra Pose
Nirlamba Paschimottanasana
  Unsupported Intense Back Stretch Pose
Nirlamba Ardha Padmottanasana
  Half Lotus Unsupported Forwards Bend Pose
Nirlamba Navasana
  Unsupported Boat Pose
Nirlamba Padma Sarvangasana
  Unsupported Whole Body Rejuvenating Lotus Pose
NiralambaPadmaShirshasana
  Hands-Free Lotus Head Stand Pose
Niralamba Padma Sirsasana
  Hands Free Lotus Headstand Pose (Arms Spread Wide Open Var.)
Nirlamba Sarvangasana
  Unsupported Whole Body Rejuvenating Pose
Nirlamba Rajakapotasana
  Unsupported King Pigeon Pose
Niralamba Sarvangasana
  Unsupported Shoulder Stand Pose I
Niralamba Sarvangasana II
  Unsupported Shoulder Stand Pose II (Prep).
Niralamba Sarvangasana II
  Unsupported Shoulder Stand Pose II
Nirlamba Sirsa Padasana
  Unsupported Feet To Head Pose
Niralamba-Shirshasana
  Hands-Free Head Stand Pose

Nirlamba Urdhva Prasarita Ekapadasana
  Unsupported One Leg Extended Forward Bend Pose
Nirlamba Utthana Hasta Padasana
  Unsupported Arms And Leg Stretch Pose
Nirlamba Vygarasana
  Unsupported Tiger stretch Pose

O

Omkarasana
  Om Pose

P

Pada Hastasana
  Hand Under Foot Pose
Pada Mayurasana
  Lotus Peacock Pose
Pada Paschima Hanumanasana
  Lord Hanuman Pose – Foot Touching The Back
Pada Shirsha Urdhva Dhanurasana
  Foot to Head Raised Bow Pose
Padahastasana
  Feeton Hands Pose
Padangustha Chakra Bandhasana
  Tip Toe Bound Wheel Pose
Padangustha Dhanurasana
  Bid Toe Bow Pose
Padangustha Eka Pada Sirsasana
  Tip Toes Balance Foot Behind The Head Pose
Padangustha Himalayasana
  One Arm Holding The big Toe – Mount Himalaya Pose
Padangustha Kapotasana
  Tip Toe Pigeon Pose
Padangustha Kapatasana
  Tip Toe Pigeon Pose

Padangustha Parivrtta Hanumasana
  Revolved Lord Hanuman Pose – With One Arm Hold
  The Big Toe
Padangustha Setu Bandasana Pose
  Tiptoe Bridge Pose
Padapaschima Rajakapotasana
  Feet Touching The Back King Pigeon
Padma Bhujangangasana
  Lotus/ King Cobra Pose
Padma Bhujangasana
  Lotus Cobra Pose
Padma Halasana
  Lotus Plough Pose
Padma Mayurasana
  Lotus Peacock Pose
Padma Sarvangasana
  Lotus Shoulder Stand Pose
Padma Sayanasana
  Lotus Couch Pose
Padma Setubandhasana
  Lotus Bridge Pose
Padma Shirshasana
  Lotus Pose Headstand
Parighasana
  Gate Pose
Paripurna Bhujangasana
  Complete Cobra Pose
Paripurna Bogarasana
  Sage Bogar Pose – Complete
Paripurna Eka Pada Rajakapotasana
  Complete King Pigeon Pose – One Leg
Paripurna Dhanurasana
  Complete Bow Pose
Paripurna Hanumasana
  Lord Hanuman Pose – Complete
Paripurna Korakarasana
  Sage Korakar Pose – Complete

Paripurna Marichyasana
  Sage Marichi Pose – Complete
Paripurna Matsyendrasana I
  Full Spinal Twist Lord of the Fishes
Paripurna Matsyendrasana II
  Complete Lord of the Fishes Pose
Paripurna-Navasana
  Complete Boat Pose
Paripurna Nindra Dhanurasana
  Standing Full Bow Pulling Pose
Paripurna Paschimottanasana
  Complete Back stretch Pose
Paripurna Raja Kapotasana
  Complete King Pigeon Pose
Paripurna Utthita Vrschikasana
  Elevated Scorpion – Complete
Paripurna Vajrasana
  Thunder Bolt Pose – Complete
Paripurna Vamadevasana
  Sage Vamadeva Pose – Complete
Paripurna Vrschikasana
  Raised Lotus In Scorpion Pose
Parivid Pada Bhujangasana
  Twined Legs Snake Pose
Parivrtta Ardha Chandrasana
  Revolved Half Moon
Parivrtta Adho Mukha Shvanasana
  Revolved Downward Facing Dog
Parivrtta Baddha Ardha Chandrasana
  Revolved Bound Half Moon Pose
Parivrtta Baddha Trikonasa
  Revolved Bound Triangle Pose
Parivrtta Baddhapada Uttanasana
  Bound Legs Twisted Forward Bend Pose
Parivrtta Eka Pada Badha Hasta Uttanasana
  Revolved One Leg Hand Binding Intense
  Stretch Pose

Parivrtta Eka Pada Koundinyasana
  Revolved One Leg Sage Koundinya Pose
Parivrtta Hanumasana
  Revolved Lord Hanuman Pose
Parivrtta Janu Sirsasana/ Shirshasana
  Revolved Head to Knee Pose
Parivrtta Natarajasana
  Shiva Twist
Parivrtta Parsva Konasana
  Revolved Side Angle Pose
Parivrtta Parsvakonasana /Parshvakonasana
  Revolved Side Angle Pose
Parivrtta Parsvottanasana
  Revolved Side Stretch Pose
Parivrtta Paschimottanasana
  Revolved Seated Forward Bend
Parivrtta Prasarita Padottanasana
  Revovled Wide Angle Forward Bend Pose
Parivrtta Trikonasana
  Revolved Triangle
Parivrtta Trikonasana
  Revolved Triangle Pose Variation
Parivrtta Parsvakonasana
  Revolved Side Angle Pose (Prayer Hand Namaskar Variation)
Parivrtta Utkatasana
  Twisted Powerful Pose
Parivrtta Utkatasana
  Revolved Chair Pose
Parivrtta Upavistha Konasana
  Revolved Open Angle Seated Forward Bend
Parivrtta Uttana Anjaliasana
  Revolved Standing Forward Bend Prayer Pose
Parivrtta Uttanasana
  Revovled Intense Standing Forward Bend
Parivrtta Utthita Pada Hasthasana
  Revolved – Extended Hand To Feet Pose

Parivrttaikapada-Shirshasana
　Revolving One Leg Head Stand Pose
Parivrrtapada Baddha Konasana
　Twisted Feet Bound Angle Pose
Parshva Halasana
　Side Plough Pose
Parshva Kukkutasana
　Side Cock Pose
Parshva Padma Sarvangasana
　Side Lotus Shoulder Stand Pose
Parshva Pindasana
　Side Embryo Pose
Parshva Salamba Shirshasana
　Supported Side Head stand Pose
Parshva Sarvangasana
　Side Shoulder Stand Pose
Parshva Shavasana
　Side Corpse Pose
Parshva Shirshasana
　Side Head Pose
Parshva Padma Shirshasana
　Side Lotus Pose Headstand
Parshva Upavishta Konasana
　Side Seated Angle Pose
Parsva Ardha Bakasana
　Side Crane Pose
Parsva Bakasana
　Side Crane Pose
Parsva Dandasana
　Twisted Staff Pose
Parsva Dhanurasana
　Side Bow
Parsva Halasana
　Sideways Plough Pose
Parsva Karnapidasana
　Sideways Knee-to-Ear Pose
Parsva Konasana
　Side Angle Pose

Parsva Kukkutasana
  Side Cock Pose
Parsva Padma Parvatasana
  Lateral Lotus Mountain Pose
Parsva Pindasana in Halasana
  Sideways Embryo Plough Pose
Parsva Upavistha Konasana
  Side Seated Angle
Parsva Urdhva Padmasana in Sirsasana I
  Sideways Upward Lotus in Headstand I
Parsva Urdhva Padmasana in Sirsasana II
  Sideways Upward Lotus in Headstand II
Parsva Urdhva Padmasana in Sarvangasana I
  Sideways Upward Lotus in Shoulder Stand I
Parsva Vamadevasana
  Sage Vamadeva Pose – Flanked
Parsva Sarvangasana
  Sideways Shoulder Stand
Parsva Sirsasana I
  Sideways Headstand I
Parsva Sirsasana II
  Sideways Headstand II
Parsva Veerabhadrasana
  Sideways Warrior Verrabhadra Pose
Parsva Vrksanasa
  Flanked Tree Pose
Parsva Yoga Mudrasana
  Side-Bending Yogic Seal
Parsavasana
  Side Stretch Pose
Parsvaika Pada Sarvangasana I
  One-Legged Sideways Shoulder Stand I
Parshvakakasana
  Side Crow Pose
Parsvottanasana/Parshvottanasana
  Side Intense Stretch Pose Prep

Parshvottanasana
  Intense Side Stretch Pose (Interlocking Fingers Variation)
Parshvottanasana
  Side Intense Stretch Pose/ Pyramid
Paryankasana
  Bed Pose
Pasasana
  Noose Pose
Paschimatanasana
  Seated Forward Bend/ Back Stretch Pose
Paschimottanasana Namaskar
  Forward Bend with Hands in Prayer Pose
Pashasana
  Noose Pose
Pavana Muktasana
  Wind Relieving Pose
Patanjaliasana
  Sage Patanjali Pose
Patanvrkshasana
  Toppling Tree Pose
Peraiyasana
  Crescent Moon Pose
Phalakasana
  Plank
Pincha Janu Marichyasna
  Chin To Knee Sage Marichi
Pincha Mayurasana
  Peacock Feather Pose
Pinda–Shirshasana
  Embryo Lotus Pose Headstand
Pindasana
  Embryo Pose
Pindasana in Halasana
  Embryo Plough Pose
Pindasana in Sirsasana I
  Embryo Pose in Headstand I

Prapada-Matsyendrasana
  Spinal Twist in Tiptoe Pose
Prapada-Paryankasana
  Tiptoe Couch Pose
Prapada-Setu-Bhandasana
  Tiptoe Bridge-Forming Pose
Prapadasana
  Tiptoe Pose
Prapardasana
  Tiptoe Pose
Prasaritha Pada Halasana
  Feet Spread Out Plough Pose
Prasarita Eka Pada Sirsa Padasana
  One Leg Stretched Out Foot Touching Head Pose
Prasarita Pada Paschimottanasana
  Feet Spread Out Forward Bend Pose
Prasarita Pada Rajakapotasana
  King Pigeon Pose – One Leg Stretched Out
Prasaritha Pada Nirlamba Halasana
  Feet Spread Out Unsupported Plough Pose
Prasarita Padottanasana
  Revolved Wide Angle Forward Bend
Prasarita Padottasana I
  Wide Angle Standing Forward Bend I
Prasarita Padottasana II
  Wide Angle Standing Forward Bend II
Prasarita Padottasana III
  Wide Angle Standing Forward Bend III
Prasarita Padottasana IV
  Wide Angle Standing Forward Bend IV
Punnakeesarasana
  Sage Punnakeesar Pose
Purna-Chakrasana
  Full Wheel Pose
Purna Matsyendrasana
  Sage Matsyendra's Pose – Complete (Lotus Variation)
Purna Salabasana
  Full Locust Pose

Purna Ustrasana
  Camel Pose – Full
Purna Vamadevasana
  Sage Vamadeva Pose – Full
Purvottanasana
  Intense Front Body Stretch
Purvottana Padma Sarvangasana
  Intense Front Body stretching & Rejuvenating Lotus Pose

Q

R

Raja Bhujangasana
  King Cobra Pose
Raja Hanumanasana
  King Leg-Split Pose Dedicated to Hanuman
Raja Kapotasana
  King Pigeon Pose
Raja Kurmasana
  King Tortoise Pose
RajaValakhilyasana
  Kingly Pose of the Heavenly Spirits
Romarishi Asana
  Sage Romarishi Pose
Ruchikasana
  Pose of the Sage Ruchika

S

Salabasana /Salabhasana
  Locust Pose
Salamba Angula Sirsasana
  Thumbs Supported Headstand Pose
Salamba Bhujangasana
  Sphinx
Salamba Navasana
  Supported Boat Pose

Salambha Padma Shirshasana
  Supported Lotus Head Stand (Forearm Touch Var.)
Salamba Padma
  Supported Lotus Headstand Pose
Salamba Parsva Veerabhadrasana
  Sideways Warrior Verrabhadra Pose –Supported
Salamba Pindasana
  Supported Embryo Pose
SalambaSarvangasana
  Supported Shoulder Stand Pose
Salambha Shirshasana
  Supported Head Stand (Reverse Tripod Forearms Touch Var.)
Salamba Shirshasana
  Supported Headstand Pose (Reverse Tripod Var.)
Salamba Sarvangasana I
  Supported Shoulder Stand I
Salamba Sarvangasana II
  Supported Shoulder Stand II
Salamba Shirshasana/ Sirsasana
  Tripod Supported Head Stand Pose
Samakonasana
  Even Angle Pose/ Even Angle Pose
Sankarasana
  Yogi Sankarar Pose
Sarpasana
  Snake
Sarvangasana
  Shoulder Stand Pose
Sasangasana
  Rabbit Pose
Sattaimuni Asana
  Sage Sattaimuni Pose
Savasana
  Corpse Pose
Sayanasana
  Couch Pose

Setu Bandha
  Bridge Pose
Setu-Bandha-Parshva-Sarvangasana
  Bridge Shoulder Stand Pose
Setu Bandha Sarvangasana
  Bridge Pose
Setu Bandha Sarvangasana
  Bridge Pose (Prep.)
Setu Bandhasana
  Bridge Forming Pose
Shalabhasana
  Locust
Shashankasana
  Hare Pose
Shatkonasana
  Six Triangle Pose
Shavasana
  Corpse Pose
Simhasana
  Lion Pose
Shirsha-Pada-Eka-Adho-Mukha-Vrkshasana
  Foot to Head One-Hand Hand stand Pose
Shirsha Padasana
  Foot to Head Pose (Prep.)
Shirsha Padasana
  Foot to Head Pose
Shirshasana
  Head Pose
Shitali-Kumbahka
  Cooling Retention of Inhalation
Shivathandavasana
  Lord Shiva's Dancing Pose
Sirsa Pada Eka Hasta Adho Mukha Vrksasana
  Foot to Head One Hand Handstand Pose
Sirsa Pada Mayurasana
  Head To Feet Peacock Pose
Sirsa Pada Natarajasana
  Foot To Head Dancer's Pose

Sira Padasana
  Feet to Head Pose
Sirsasana
  Headstand (Prep)
Sirsasana I
  Headstand I
Sirsasana II
  Enlightened Headstand Pose Buddha
Sirsasana III
  Headstand III
Sirsasana IV
  Headstand IV
Sirspada Laghu Dhanurasana
  Feet To Head Little Bow Pose
Sirsapadasana
  Feet To Head Pose
Siddhasana
  Accomplished/ Adept's Pose
Sivanandasana
  Yogi Sivananda's Pose
Skandasana
  Pose of the Lord Skanda/ Pose Dedicated to the God of War
Squatting
dm641
Sukha Matsyasana
  Easy Fish Pose
Supta Baddha Konasana
  Reclining Bound Angle Pose/ Supine Bound Angle
Supta Bhekasana
  Reclining Frog Pose
Supta Dwipada Danasana
  Supine Yogi's Meditating Stick Pose – Both Arms
Supta Hastha Padottanasana
  Reclined Intense Leg Stretch Pose
Supta Konasana
  Reclining Wide Angle Pose

Supta Koormasana
  Reclined Tortoise Pose
Supta Koorma
  Anjaliasana Reclined Tortoise Prayer Pose
Supta Madhyasana
  Reclining Waist Pose
Supta Padangusthasana I
  Reclining Big Toe Pose I
Supta Padangusthasana II
  Reclining Big Toe Pose II
Supta Virasana
  Reclining Hero Pose
Supta Matsyendrasana
  Knee Down Twist
Supta Padangusthasana
  Supine Hand To Toe
Supta Vajrasana
  Supine Thunderbolt Pose
Supta-Virasana
  Reclining Hero Pose
Supta-Trivikramasama
  Reclining Vishnu Pose
Surya Namaskarasana
  Sun Salutation Pose
Surya-Namskara-Adho-Mukha-Svanasana
  Sun salutation –Downward Facing Dog Pose
Surya-Namskara-Ashtanga-Namaskara
  Sun Salution –Eight-Point Bow Pose
Surya-Namskara-Ashva-Sanchalanasana
  Sun Salutation –Equestrian Pose
Surya-Namskara-Ashva-Sanchalanasana
  Sun Salutation – Equestrian Pose
Surya-Namskara-Chaturanga-Dandasana
  Sun Salutation –Plank Pose
Surya-Namskara-Hasta-Uttanasana
  Sun Salutation – Raided Hands Pose
Surya-Namskara-Pranamasana
  Sun Salutation – Prayer Pose

Surya-Namaskara-Bhujangasana
 Sun Salutation– Cobra Pose
Surya-Namskara-Uttanasana
 Sun Salutation –Intense Stretch Pose
Sucirandhrasana
 Threading the Needle
Sukha Chakorasna
 Comfortable Partridge Pose
Sukha-Garbha-Pindasana
 Easy Embryo in the Womb Pose
Sukha-Matsyasana
 Easy Fish Pose
Sukha-Matsyendrasana
 Easy Spinal Twist
Sukha-Rajakapotasana
 Easy King Pigeon Pose
Sukha-Supta-Kurmasana
 Easy Sleeping Tortoise Pose
Sukhasana
 Easy Pose
Sundaranandar Asana
 Sage Sundaranandar Pose
Svanasana
 Dog Tilt Pose
Sutra-Neti
 String Neti/ Nasal Cleansing

T

Table
 Table Pose
Tadasana
 Mountain Pose
Tadasana
 Mountain Pose Variation
Tadasana Urdhva Baddha Hastasana
 Mountain Pose with Bound Hands

Tadasana Urdhva Hastasana
  Mountain Pose with Arms Overhead
Tadasana Samasthiti
  Mountain Pose/ Steady Standing
Tarasana
  Star Pose
Thavaliasana
  Frog Pose
Thirumoolararasana Sage
  Thirumoolar Pose
Thiruvikramasana
  Lord Shiva's Terrific Dance Pose
Tiriang Mukhottonasana
  Standing Intense Backbend Pose
Triang Mukhaikapada Paschimottanasana
  Three-Limbed Forward Bend
Tiriang Mukhottanasana
  Intense Backbend Stretch
Tiriend Pada Akarna Dhanurasana
  Crossed Leg Archer Pose
Tittibhasana/ Titibhasana
  Firefly Pose
Trikonasana
  Triangle Pose (Preparation)
Trikonasana
  Triangle Pose/ Five Pointed Star
Trikonasana
  Triangle Pose (Variation)
Tiriang Baddha Pada Natarajasana
  Intense Backbend Bound Leg/ Feet Shiva's Dancing
  Pose
Tiryaka Tadasana
  Swaying Tree Pose
Tolasana
  Scale Pose
Tryanga-Mukhaikapada-Paschimatanasana
  Three-Limbed Facing One-Foot Back Stretch
  Pose

U

Ubhaya Padangushtasana
  Big Toe Pose
Uddhiyana Marjaryasana
  Abdominal Cat Lift A
Uddiyana Bandha
  Abdominal Lock
Upavista/Upavistha Konasana I
  UpwardFacing Open Angle Pose
Upavista/Upavistha Konasana II
  Open Angle Seated Forward Bend
Upavistha Konasana in Adho Mukha Vrksasana
  Open-Angle Pose in Handstand
Upavistha Prapadasana
  Crouching Tiptoe Pose
Upavistha Yoga Mudra
  Seated Yoga Seal
Urdhva Ardha Padma Paschimottanasana
  Upward Facing Forward Bend
Urdhva Dandasana in Adho Mukha Vrksasana
  Full Arm Balance
Urdhva Dandasana
  Upward/ Inverted Staff Pose
Urdhva Dandasana II
  Upward/ Inverted Staff Pose II
Urdhva Dandasana III
  Upward/ Inverted Staff Pose III
Urdhva-Dhanurasana
  Upward/ Raised Bow Pose
Urdhva Eka Hastha Padma Bhujangasana
  One Arm Stretched Up Lotus Cobra Pose
Urdhva Hastha Virasana
  Raised Arms Warrior Pose
Urdhva Hastha Yoga Nidrasana
  Arms Raised Up Yogi's Sleeping Pose

Urdhva Hastasana in Virasana
 Hero Pose with Arms Overhead.
Urdhva Hastasana in Padmanasana
 Lotus Pose with Arms Overhead
Urdhva Kukkutasana
 Raised/ Upward Cock Pose
Urdhva Matsyasana
 Raised Fish Pose
Urdhva Mayurasana
 Inverted Peacock Pose
Urdhva Mukha Makarasana
 Upward Facing Crocodile Pose
Urdhva Mukha Moola Bhandhasana
 Upward Facing Perineal Contraction Pose
Urdhva Mukha Paksiyasana
 Upward Facing Bird Pose
Urdhva Mukha Paschimatanasana I
 Upward Facing Back Stretch Pose
Urdhva Muka Paschimatanasana II
 Upward Facing Back Stretch Pose II
Urdhva Mukha Paripruna Nindra Nindra Dhanurasana
 Upward Facing Standing Full Bow
 Pulling Pose
Urdhva Mukha Prasarita Padottanasana
 Upward Facing Wide Legs Forward Bend Pose
Urdhva Mukha Paschimottanasana I
 Upward Facing Forward Bend (Var.)
Urdhva Mukha Paschimottanasana II
 Upwardfacing Forward Bend II
Urdhva Mukha Svanasana
 UpwardFacing Dog
Urdhva Mukha Utthita Dwipada Viparita Danasana
 Upward Facing Elevated Both Legs
 Inverted Staff Pose
Urdhva Mukha Eka Hasta Padangustha Nukasana
 Upward Facing One Leg BigToe Boat
 Pose

Urdhva Mukha Kailiasana
  Upward Facing Goddess Kali Pose
Urdhva Mukha Korakarasana
  Upward Facing Sage Korakar Pose
Urdhva Mukha Niralamba Bhujangasana
  Upward Facing Unsupported Cobra Pose
Urdhva Mukha Niralamba Sarpasana
  Upward Facing Unsupported Snake Pose
Urdhva Mukha Svanasana
  Upward Facing Dog Pose
Urdhva Pada Brahmacharyasana
  Upward Tending Celebate Pose
Urdhva Padma Mayurasana
  Inverted Lotus Peacock Pose
Urdhva Padma Padma Hamsasana
  Upward Tending Lotus Swan Pose
Urdhva Padma Salabasana
  Raised Lotus Locust Pose
Urdhva Padma Vrschikasana
  Upward/ Raised Scorpion Pose
Urdhva Padmasana Upward Tending Lotus Pose
Urdhva Padmasana
  Upward Lotus Pose
Urdhva Padmasana in Adho Mukha Vrksasana
  Inverted Lotus in Handstand
Urdhva Padmasana in Baddha Hasta Sirsasana
  Upward Lotus in Bound Hand Headstand
Urdhva Padmasana in Mukta Hasta Sirsasana
  Upward Lotus in Free-Hand Headstand
Urdhva Padmasana in Sarvangasana
  Upward Lotus in Shoulder Stand I
Urdhva Padmasana in Sirsasana I
  Upward Lotus in Headstand I Front
Urdhva Padmasana in Sirsasana II
  Upward Lotus in Headstand II
Urdhva Padmasana in Sirsasana III
  Upward Lotus in Headstand III

Urdhva Paschimottanasana
  Upward Tending Intense Back Stretch Pose
Urdhva Prasarita Eka Padasana
  One Leg Extended Forward Bend Pose
Urdhva Salabasana
  Raised Locust Pose
Urdhva Upavista Konasana
  Upward Facing Open Angle Pose
Urdhva Upavista Paschimottanasana
  Upward-Facing Open Angle Forward Bend I
Urdhva Upavishta Konasana
  Upright Seated Angle
Urdhva Uttanasana
  Upward Forward Fold
Ustrasana
  Camel Pose
Utkata Konasana
  Goddess Squat
Utkatasana
  Chair Pose/Fierce Pose
Uttanasana
  Standing Forward Fold
Utripada Padma Sirsasana
  Tripod Headstand Lotus Pose
Utripada Sirsa Baddha Konasana
  Bound Angle Tripod Headstand Pose
Utripada Sirsa Samakonasana
  Tripod Headstand Same Angle Pose
Uttanasana
  Intense Stretch Pose (Interlocking Fingers Variation)
Uttana Bogarasana
  Triangle Pose
Uttana Padasana
  Intense Leg Stretch
Uttana Padma Mayurasana
  Intense Lotus Peacock
Uttanasana
  Standing Forward Bend

Uttanasana
  Intense Stretch Pose Stork (Variation)
Uttanasana
  Intense Stretch Pose (Cross Forearm Grab Feet Variation)
Utthana Merudandasana
  Intense Backbend Pose
Utthita Ashwa Sanchalanasana
  High Lunge
Utthita Baddha Hastha Janu Sirsasana
  Standing Bound Arms Head Between Knees
Utthita Baddha Konasana
  Lifted Cobbler Pose
Utthita Bhujangasana
  Standing Cobra Pose
Utthita Dwipada Sirsasana
  Lifted Feet Behind The Head Pose
Utthita Dwipada Viparita Dandasana
  Elevated Both Legs Inverted Staff Pose
Utthita Dwipada Vrstasana
  Raised Up Feet Spread out Resting On The Arms Pose
Utthita Eka Pada Adho Muka Svanasana
  One Leg Raised Up Downward Facing Dog Pose
Utthita Eka Pada Bakasana
  One Leg Raised Up Crane Pose
Utthita Eka Pada Chakrasana
  Dwipada Viparita Dandasana One Leg Raised Up Wheel Pose
Utthita Eka Pada Cibi Januasana
  Standing Chin To Knee Pose
Utthita Eka pada Paripurna Masyendrasana
  Sage Matsyendra Pose Complete
Utthita Eka Pada Paschimottanasana
  Raised Up Leg & Back Stretch Pose
Utthita Eka pada Sirsasana
  Lifted Foot Behind The Head Pose
Utthitha Eka Pada Viparita Dandasana
  One Leg Rasied Up Inverted Staff Pose

Utthita Eka Pada Yoga Dandasana
  One Leg Stretched Up Yogi's Meditating Stick Pose
Utthita Ganda Bherundasana
  Extended Formidable Face Pose
Utthita Padmasana
  Lofted Lotus Pose
Utthita Hastha Pada Uttanasana
  Extended Hand To Foot Stretch Pose
Utthita Hasta Padangusthaana
  Extended Hand To Big Toe Pose
Utthita Hasta Padangusthasana
  Standing Hand to Big Toe Pose (Variation)
Utthita Koormasana
  Raised Tortoise Pose
Uttana Padasana
  Extended Leg Pose
Utthita Parivrtta Baddha Padasana
  Raised & Revolved Bound Leg Stretch Pose
Utthita Parsvakonasana
  Extended Side Angle Pose
UtthitaParshvasahita
  Standing Leg Going to the Side Pose
Utthita Purna Salabasana
  Elevated Full Locust Pose
Utthita Raja Vrschikasana
  Elevated King Scorpion Pose
Utthita Supta Padangusthasana
  Extended Supine Hand To Toe
Utthita Svanasana
  Extended Dog Pose
Utthita Trikonasana
  Extended Triangle Pose
Utthita Tittibhasana
  Standing Firefly Pose
Utthita-Vayu-Muktyasana
  Standing Wind Relieving Pose Variation
Utthita Vayu Muktyasana
  Standing Wind Relieving Pose

Utthita Tittibhasana
  Standing Firefly Pose (Full Insect Pose)
Utthita Tittibhasana
  Standing Firefly Pose (Binding Interlocking Fingers Variation)
Utthita Vrschikasana
  Elevated Scorpion Pose

V

Vaasamni
  Asana Sage Vaasamuni Pose
Vajrasana
  Thunderbolt Pose
Vakrasana
  Crooked Pose
Valakhilyasana
  Pose of the Heavenly Spirits/ Divine Spirit Pose
Valgulasana
  Vishnu Bat Pose
Valmiki Asana
  Sage Valmiki Pose
Vamadevasana I
  Pose Dedicated to the Sage Vamadeva
Vamadevasana II
  Pose Dedicated to the Sage Vamadeva
Vamana Nauli
  Left Side Isolation
Vasisthasana
  Pose Dedicated to the Sage Vasistha
Vatayanasana
  Horse Pose / Sea Horse Pose
Vatayanasana
  Horse Pose (Namaste Palm Prayer Variation)
Vayu-Muktyasana
  Wind-Relieving Pose
Veerabhasdrasana Warrior
  Veerabhadra Pose

Veerasana
　Warrior Pose
Veerastambanasana
　Warrior Veerastamban Pose
Vibhakta Vrschikasana
　Symmetical Scorpion Pose
Viparita Pindasana
　Inverted Embryo In The Womb Pose
Viparita Bhekasana
　Inverted Frog Pose
Viparita Dwipada Anjaliasana
　Inverted – Both Legs Prayer Pose
Viparita Dwipada Baddhasana
　Inverted Bound Legs Pose
Viparita Garbapindasana
　Inverted Embryo In The Womb Pose
Viparita Karani Mudra
　Inverted Lake Seal
Viparita Karnapida Urdhva Padmasana
　Inverted Ear Pressure Raised Up Lotus Pose
Viparita Koormasana
　Inverted Tortoise Pose
Viparita Raja Koormasana
　Inverted King Tortoise Pose
Viparita Shalabhasana
　Inverted Locust Pose
Viparita Titibha Anjali Asana
　Inverted Firefly Prayer Pose
Viparita Titibhasana
　Inverted Firefly Pose
Viparita Virabhadrasana
　Reverse Warrior
Vipateetha Salabasana
　Inverted Locust Pose
Vira Parampara I
　Hero Series I
Vira Parampara II
　Hero Series II

Vira Parampara III
  Hero Series III
Vira Parampara IV
  Hero Series IV
Vira Parampara V
  Hero Series V
Vira Parampara VI
  Hero Series VI
Vira Parampara VII
  Hero Series VII
Vira Parampara VIII
  Hero Series VIII
Vira Parampara IX
  Hero Series IX
Vira Parampara X
  Hero Series X
Vira Tolasana
  Hero Scale Pose
Virabhadra Mudra
  Warrior Seal
Virabhadrasana I
  Warrior Pose
Virabhadrasana II
  Warrior Pose II
Viranchyasana I
  Pose Dedicated to Viranchi (Brahma)
Virasana
  Hero Pose
Vishnu-Devanandasana
  Yogi Vishnu-Devanda's Pose
Vishnu Devanandasana
  Vishnu Devananda's Pose (Variation)
Visvamitrasana/ Vishvamitrasana
  Pose Dedicated to the Sage Visvamitra
Viswamitasana
  Sage Viswamitra Pose
Vrksasanas
  Tree Pose

Vrksasana Vari
  Tree Pose (Vari Leaning Over)
Vrschika Anjaliasana
  Scorpion Prayer Pose
Vrschikasana
  Scorpion Pose (Variation)
Vrschikasana
  Scorpion Pose
Vrschikasana II
  Scorpion Pose II (Feet to Head)
Vyaghrasana
  Tiger Pose

Y

Yajnasana
  Christ's Cross Pose
Yoganidrasana
  Yogic Sleep
Yoga Mudra /Mudrasana
  Yogic Seal
Yoga Nidrasana
  Yogi's Sleeping Pose
Yoganandasana
  Yogi Yogananda Pose
Yogasana
  Yoga Pose
Yudhasana
  Fighting Warrior Pose

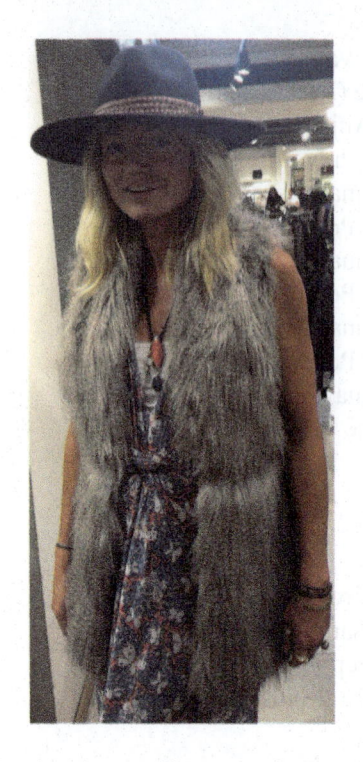

Sarah Tucker is a best selling novelist, award winning journalist, broadcaster and travel writer. Currently studying to be a sports psychologist and a qualified yoga instructor, she takes yoga workshops in Surrey and SW London as well as overseas.

Further details
www.atozenoftravel.com
www.atozenofyoga.com
www.atozenoflife.com
twitter @madasatucker
www.sarahtucker.info
email info@atozenoftravel.com

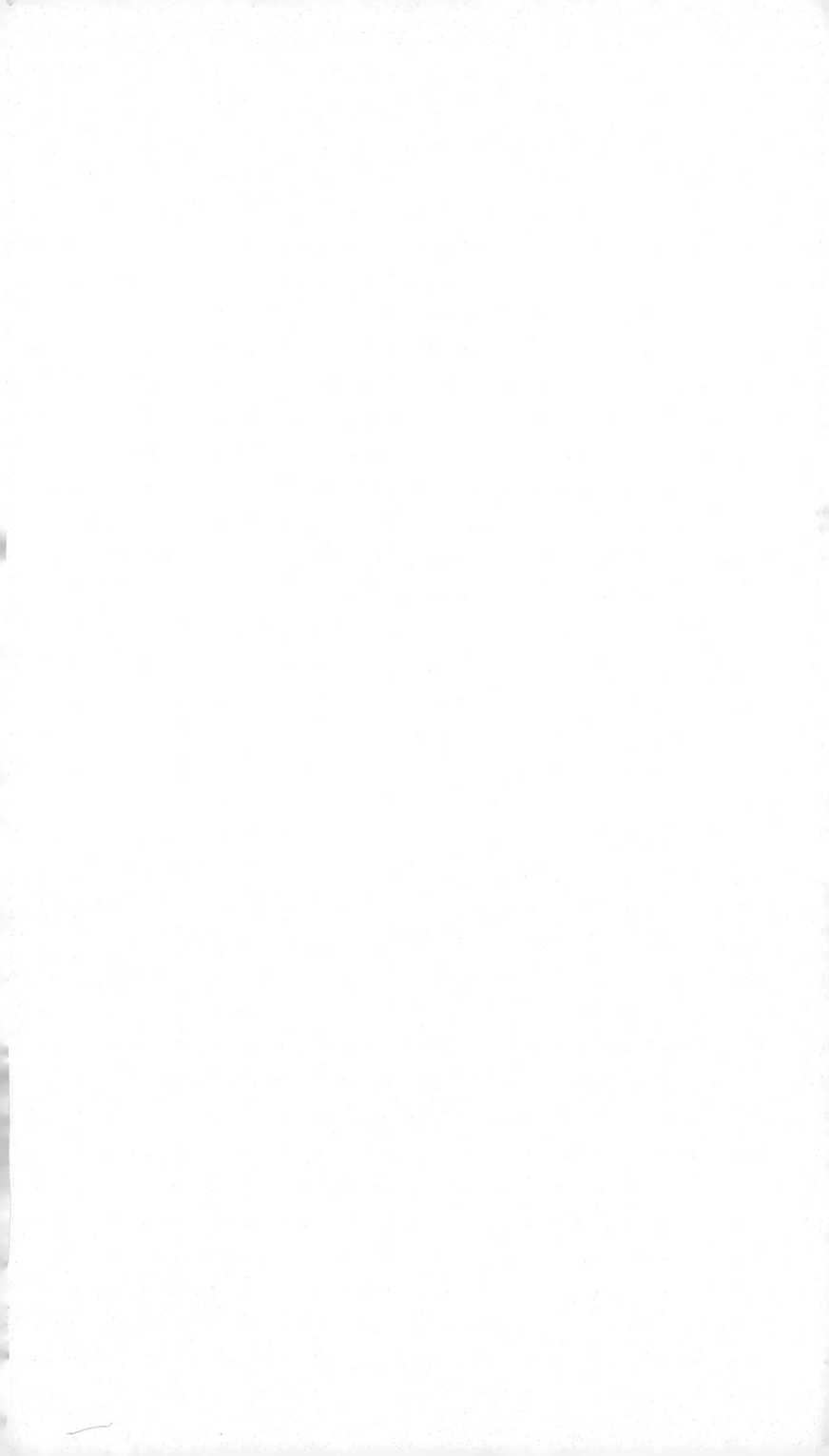